TRANSFORM YOUR LIFE WITH INTERMITTENT FASTING FOR WOMEN OVER 50

5 MAJOR PRINCIPLES TO HELP YOU LOSE WEIGHT AND REVITALIZE YOUR BODY

RILEY CALDWELL

CONTENTS

INTRODUCTION

Are you a middle-aged woman looking to slim down? If you tried everything, from dieting to exercising, and nothing seems to work, you're not alone. Many middle-aged women find that old tricks no longer work when it comes to staying healthy and slim. Reduce calories? You won't lose weight! Start working out more? That doesn't seem to work, either. It appears as though no matter what you do, you're seeing no improvement.

But wait, don't lose faith just yet! I have a solution that might help, and it's proven to be effective in helping women over 50 lose weight. That solution is called intermittent fasting.

If you've just now heard about intermittent fasting, welcome to the club! Intermittent fasting is a lifestyle built upon the backing of research studies that showed how the modern lifestyle of eating sugary foods and having meals spread out the entire day depletes health and leads to weight gain.

Wait, but isn't having multiple smaller meals exactly what you were told to do to slim down? In this book, you'll learn about the many misconceptions about healthy eating, or rather rules that no longer apply. You'll learn why you should stop doing the following:

- Eat breakfast as soon as you get up.
- Have five or more meals from early morning to late evening.
- Cut back on meat and fats if you're trying to lose weight.
- And more!

The science behind intermittent fasting shows us all the intricate layers of the human metabolic system and, more importantly, how to get your metabolic system to start burning fat.

What better way to master intermittent fasting than learn from someone who succeeded with it? I am proud to say that I have been fasting for five whole years. During this time, I managed to regain my mental clarity and muscle tone, all while lowering body fat. If there's one thing I'd recommend for anyone passionate about health and wellness, this would be it.

I wrote this book intending to provide a thorough understanding of what intermittent fasting is. I want to show you exactly how it works and how you can benefit from it. You need this book if:

- **You're a middle-aged woman who is struggling to lose weight.** Did you think that you can't lose weight simply because of your age? Wrong! This book will show you what makes your body unique in this stage of life and what you can do to better adjust to these changes. Middle-aged women are proven to be able to exercise and lose weight just fine. Need motivation? Look up image results for "Fit women over 50," and you'll be amazed at just how much women can build themselves up. If you've deemed yourself too old to be fit and look great, think again. You can follow in the footsteps of Mariah Carey, Jane Fonda, Julia Roberts, Jennifer Anniston, Jennifer Lopez, and many more ladies who pride themselves on a healthy lifestyle. No expensive treatments, no life-threatening surgeries. You alone, your willpower, and a little bit of knowledge are enough to start making a change. But before you're able to do that, you need to get to know your body. You need to learn about your metabolism and how it's different from what it used to be. With this knowledge, you'll have a better understanding of why classic rules of healthy eating and living no longer apply and why it's necessary to try an innovative approach.

- **You wish to regain vitality and adopt a new lifestyle that's been proven to promote longevity.** A middle-aged woman can be slim, good-looking, vital, and healthy. You don't need to be a Hollywood star! You don't even need to allocate a budget. All you need to do is learn about fasting. Fasting is, in fact, a body's natural state, and it's been with mankind since its inception. Yet, in the past 100 years, our lifestyles became quite distant from how our bodies were initially designed to operate. We no longer eat because we need to but because we want to. We eat out of boredom, because everyone else is eating, or because it's time to eat. Not anymore! This book will teach you to view food as an ally in maintaining health and not as a necessity, coping mechanism, or chore. I'll help you develop a healthier relationship with food so that you can start listening to your

body and give it the nutrition that it truly
needs.

- **You want to finally overcome depression,
  dissatisfaction with your body and looks, and
  drastic mood swings that occur as a result of
  hormonal imbalance in your body.** Did you
  know that diet has a direct impact on your
  hormonal balance? Mood swings and
  depression have never correlated with obesity
  and insulin resistance more than in the past few
  decades. Packaged foods, take-out, sugary
  beverages, salty snacks, and sweets are
  poisoning your body from the inside. This book
  will show you what unhealthy eating has to do
  with emotional and hormonal imbalances.
  You'll learn how to use fasting as a way for your
  body's hormonal systems to regain natural
  balance. Fasting has been proven to help
  women improve PCOS, depression, mood
  swings, diabetes, cardiovascular problems, and
  much more!

Why spend another minute randomly snacking while
your cells stew in insulin, which ultimately feeds your
fat cells while leaving your tissues and organs starving
for nutrients? No more disappointing fads. It's time to
try a lifestyle that works. Decide now that you wish to

change your lifestyle and eat a wholesome diet that replenishes your body from the inside out while enjoying all the proven health benefits of fasting.

Hurry up and head to Chapter 1, where you'll learn about intermittent fasting and all the amazing ways in which it helps heal your body and lose weight!

1

WHAT IS INTERMITTENT FASTING, AND HOW DOES IT WORK?

Long gone are the days when you just cut down on carbs and shed weight effortlessly. As we mature, it becomes apparent that our bodies require a lot more effort and care to stay fit and healthy. If you feel frustrated by the inability to lose weight, millions of women around the world feel your pain.

Most women share your struggle, as their bodies change over time faster than they can keep up. Yet, these changes can weigh heavy once they begin to interfere with the lifestyle that we want. If your shape keeps you from enjoying your life and wearing what you love while the declining health chips away at enjoying work and social life, that means you need a change.

WHY IS IT MORE DIFFICULT TO LOSE WEIGHT AFTER 50?

Losing weight is challenging for different reasons. Almost every age group, both men and women, faces challenges when trying to slim down. There are many biological reasons for our metabolism slowing down. Yet, I dare say that the core reason for the struggle to lose weight lies in why you gained excess weight in the first place.

Most women are healthy and fit when they lead a healthy lifestyle without much stress and keep up a recommended activity pace for their body type.

Weight gain signals that your lifestyle is imbalanced. Sometimes, it's too little physical activity or a diet overly saturated with fats and carbs. Other times, there is an underlying health condition affecting your metabolism. Weight gain can also result from distress. Tension, depression, and daily coping with bad moods lead to less physical activity and eating more unhealthy foods.

Sadly, excess pounds are easy to gain and hard to lose. Weight loss becomes even more difficult after you turn 50. Sometimes, struggling to slim down can make you feel guilty. You might feel like your shape and health are damaged beyond repair. Many women think they can no longer improve their well-being, which is untrue. You can start to turn your physique and health for the better regardless of age. However, you first need to understand how your metabolism and fat burning are different now than in previous years. Here are several reasons why you struggle to slim down:

Less Muscle Mass

Women lose about 10% of their muscle mass by their 50th birthday. This makes burning fat more difficult since muscles are the chief calorie spenders in your body. Your muscles are now operating at a lower capacity, which reduces your overall daily calorie spending. Even if you are highly active, you burn fewer calories during the day than you used to.

Hormonal Changes

Your estrogen levels affect how stubbornly your body stores fat in areas like the hips, thighs, and belly. As your estrogen levels drop, your body stores fat more visibly. At the same time, your hunger and satiety hormones begin to fluctuate. Your appetite feels more intense than the sensation of satiety. These hormones can make you feel hungrier and less full after eating, causing you to eat more than needed. This imbalance is further complicated when eating a lot of refined sugars, which is proven to wreak havoc on the health of both genders and all age groups.

Lifestyle Changes

Adults start to live less active lifestyles as they get older. In fact, some studies show that adults spend between 60 and 80% of their time in physical inactivity (Carb Manager, 2022). If your day seems to go by so fast that you barely leave your office, you're not alone. Finding time for physical activity is a modern struggle that plagues everyone, starting with college students.

Yet, it is not only the lack of physical activity that makes weight loss more difficult. Along with lifestyle transformations come changes in your sleep cycle. Women find it progressively harder to fall asleep at reasonable hours, which is only partially due to watching late-night TV. Hormonal changes are underway, with the precious melatonin needed for quality sleep taking more effort to work than it once did.

Remember when you just went to bed and fell asleep peacefully at 10 p.m.? Hardly any adult does. Hormonal changes paired with increased daily worries and errands to keep up with can affect the hormones responsible for falling asleep. Weight loss is made much more difficult under sleep deprivation, and late-night eating only increases its effects.

Slower Resting Metabolism

The notion that metabolism slows down with age is a generally accepted one. However, recent studies indicate that metabolic rates stay steady by age 60 and then start slowing down (Carb Manager, 2022). Yet, the loss of muscle mass slows down your resting metabolic rate. This metabolic rate measures how much energy you spend while physically inactive. As the time women spend in more passive activities gradually increases over time due to career and lifestyle progression, so does our reliance on resting metabolism. The effects of the slower rate start to show more without adjusting food intake to your activity levels. With the added impact of hormonal changes, you might feel like your metabolism is slow.

Although losing weight may start to feel like an uphill battle, there are many things you can do to regain health and feel better about yourself. One of the ways to regain control of your health is to choose intermittent fasting.

INTERMITTENT FASTING CAN HELP!

Aside from being one of the most popular lifestyles in recent years, intermittent fasting is a proven way to lose weight and boost health. Unlike many other fad diets, intermittent fasting is a regimen that has been backed up by scientific research and evidence. Hundreds of studies showed the benefits of limiting eating times and adjusting food intake to our needs, taste, and lifestyle.

A part of what makes intermittent fasting so successful is that it is easy to keep up with if you learn the correct information beforehand. Planning your meals and choosing the form of fasting that matches your daily schedule increases your chances of success.

What Is Intermittent Fasting?

Intermittent fasting, despite its vast scientific underlay, is a simple concept. It is a lifestyle that consists only of taking a long, daily break from eating. This break should last at least 12 hours. People who are more experienced with this lifestyle fast for 36 hours or longer. This is called extended fasting.

To understand how intermittent fasting works, we should reflect on its origins. Long before people had consistent safety and access to regular food, they ate once or twice a day. After all, they didn't have a way of safely storing food and keeping it from perishing. They either had to hunt or spend a significant time cooking. Even later in the development of human civilization, when food became more abundant, people spent most of their day working. The modern eight- to nine-hour workday stems from labor rights efforts and technological progress. Before the late 19th century, it was common for people to work all day. They would take short breaks for lunch and be physically active from dusk to dawn. This lifestyle applied to children, adults, and seniors, with child labor only becoming illegal in 1938. People used to take long breaks between meals, with many eating only once daily. Gaining better access to food meant that people lived more comfortable lives. It potentially rid them of some of the benefits of fasting, though.

In the "fasted" state (during the times without eating), their bodies burned the energy from fat supplies for immediate spending. The more you eat, the more your body uses the energy gained from insulin, and stubborn fatty deposits remain unspent. When fasting, your insulin levels stay low, which causes your body to burn fat to obtain energy.

Intermittent fasting can help women over 50 shed weight in premenopausal or menopausal status. You will find plenty of scientific proof to back the benefits of intermittent fasting for weight loss. One of the studies that best highlights the effects of fasting on people with obesity examined 75 individuals who fasted for 12 weeks using the alternate-fast eating pattern. During their fasting days, the participants only had 500 calories in their overall nutrition. When not fasting, the participants ate as much as they wanted. There were no restrictions regarding calorie consumption or food choice (Carb Manager, 2022).

Another study that attests to the success of intermittent fasting examined the weight loss of obese women. These women fasted between 18 and 20 hours daily, limiting their meals to a four- to six-hour feeding window. This study shows the effects of time-restricted feeding, which entails consuming all of the daily calories within a short time(Carb Manager, 2022).

So, what did the results show? In the first study, participants improved health and weight regardless of gender, age, or menopausal status, the same as the second. The participants of the first study experienced an improvement in blood pressure and insulin resistance, aside from weight loss. In the second study, the participants showed similar metabolic improvements combined with successful fat reduction.

Fed and Fasted State

One of the more distinct features of this lifestyle is that it aims to train your metabolism to burn fat faster while not eating. This is done during the fasted state. While eating and hours afterward, your body spends energy digesting food and absorbing nutrients into the bloodstream and tissues. The main benefit of intermittent fasting is that it allows your body to spend more time in the fasting state, in part because it instills awareness of how much you eat during the day. Women often eat spontaneously and don't take random snacks and drinks into account. However, those are still calories, which don't get used up for energy but are instead stored in fat cells.

While in the fed state, your body functions slightly differently than without food in your belly. In the fasted state, your body needs the energy to survive. You need caloric fuel even when you sleep. Your brain, heart, lungs, and other organs burn calories for survival. Your glands spend energy to produce hormones that keep your body in a healthy balance. In the fasted state, your body derives this energy from fatty supplies. If you fast regularly and long enough, you can even lose weight while you sleep. This happens because your body burns fat to support its very functioning.

Although there are many variations of intermittent fasting, one stands out. It is the most common form of fasting and works well for an average woman with a busy lifestyle. It is the so-called 16/8 fasting. With this eating plan, you eat all of your meals within an eight-hour feeding window. This variation of intermittent fasting is proven to improve cholesterol and blood pressure, aside from reducing insulin resistance. While we will discuss other forms of intermittent fasting in this book, this is by far the most popular method that most women choose.

WHAT HAPPENS TO YOUR BODY WHEN YOU FAST?

What exactly happens in your body while you fast? Whether you're practicing intermittent fasting or time-restricted eating, the effects on your body are beneficial. The core benefit of fasting lies in the hormonal and metabolic changes that occur when you haven't eaten for some time. These changes benefit your overall health because they allow your body to break down harmful substances while absorbing the beneficial ones.

The time-restricted eating doesn't require caloric restriction or changes in your diet. This way, your fasting regimen is much more flexible and attainable. Reducing certain food groups in your diet or eliminating them is proven to make any dietary change hard to follow through. You're suddenly left with the responsibility to meal plan and shop more while having fewer eating options. On top of that, other fad diets reduce calories and set limitations on meal size. It becomes harder to cook healthy meals and measure your portions in the long run.

Fasting is among the most practical lifestyles as it triggers your body's natural healing processes:

Switch From Glucose to Ketones

When you fast, your body no longer has enough blood glucose. Your liver begins converting fats from your body into ketones to provide more energy. Ketones are an alternative to glucose, and their levels increase while you fast. Your body is burning fat much quicker, even while you sleep.

When you eat late at night and spread many meals throughout the day, your metabolic processes run much slower. Your cells don't pass through energy as efficiently as they do with ketosis, and you're constantly tired and sluggish. Furthermore, your body converts excess blood sugars into energy that feeds fat cells, increasing them in return.

Aside from burning fat, ketones improve the functioning of your cell mitochondria. These molecules are in charge of keeping cells and tissues energized and thoroughly affect both your health and metabolism. When you fast, your mitochondria operate more efficiently and spread energy throughout your body. You not only burn fat but also feel better rested, more clear-minded, and more energized.

Wait. Why are we suddenly talking about mitochondria? Your weight loss and health seem to go hand-in-hand, wouldn't you agree? One of the reasons for the link between keeping weight in check and being healthy is that both require your cells to process energy. Your cells, however, gradually reduce their capacity to do so efficiently. Simply put, the more capacity your cells have to process energy, the better you feel and lose weight. After all, burning fat is an act of energy processing.

Mitochondria are parts of your cells that break down fats and carbs into energy. They're organized in networks, and their connectedness supports metabolic processes. Yet, diseased cells have fragmented mitochondria. This means that the network they create to process energy no longer exists, so excess energy remains trapped in your cells. When you fast, more energy is needed for your body to function. Mitochondria start forming networks again. They're forced to break down fat in the absence of other available energy sources. This process supports cellular health and is proven to slow down your cellular aging process.

Ketosis induced by intermittent fasting helps cells become more resistant to stress. Oxidative stress that results from hormonal imbalance, toxins injected with unhealthy foods, smoking, and sleep deprivation cause damage to the cells of your body. Each cell inside your body is affected by an unhealthy lifestyle. Over time, this damage can lead to devastating illnesses. Fasting helps prevent cellular damage by making them stronger and overall better energized.

Autophagy: Self-Eating

During fasting, the body first uses stored fat as an energy source through lipolysis, which involves breaking down triglycerides (fat molecules) into glycerol and fatty acids. When fat stores are depleted, the body enters a deeper fasting state, triggering autophagy. This process breaks down damaged cellular components to generate energy and maintain cellular balance. The onset of autophagy varies based on individual metabolism, fast duration, and health but generally occurs after several hours to a few days of fasting when glucose and glycogen levels are significantly reduced. Think of this process as keeping a fire going. What's the first thing people do when they run out of wood? They start inserting everything suitable into the fire. First, they throw in old, damaged objects and then move to the old newspaper and other clutter. With this analogy, keeping your fireplace going by burning all faulty items would soon result in a tidy-looking home.

Fasting instigates metabolic switching. When you eat, your body switches from ketones to glucose, which promotes cellular growth. When glucose is present in your blood in small doses, it sparks cellular growth, which is a good thing. Your organs and tissues heal faster, creating more mitochondria to keep your body energized. The trick with intermittent fasting, as opposed to the ketogenic diet, is in that metabolic switch. While keto has its benefits, it keeps your body in the state of ketosis long-term. As opposed to that, intermittent fasting allows your body to use two different metabolic pathways.

Circadian Rhythm: Tuning Your Inner Clock

Having better-balanced hormones helps control cortisol and cholesterol levels. These substances elevate when a person is sleep deprived, under stress, and eats too many unhealthy foods. To make things worse, these often go hand in hand. The more stressed you are, the harder it is to fall asleep, and you feel more hungry because of the hormonal imbalance. Stress triggers a vicious cycle of sleep deprivation and overeating that's hard to overcome. Fasting helps attune your biological clock, a neurophysiological mechanism that sends signals to your body and regulates activities. You start to enjoy better sleep and get quality rest during the night while feeling more awake during the day. The more rest you get, the more weight you lose in return.

HOW TO SUCCEED AT INTERMITTENT FASTING

Now, let's break that devastating misconception that you no longer have control over your weight and health past 50. No, you're not at the mercy of aging and your genetic predispositions. You still have a lot of say in your body's maturation and healing. The main reason so many women find it hard to change their lifestyle and eating habits is that it takes a lot of conscious effort while results take months to show.

Luckily, switching to intermittent fasting will yield visible improvements in how you feel throughout the day. A well-implemented fasting regimen will make you feel more energized. Even before shedding pounds, you'll notice that you sleep better and have less joint and muscle pain. Your skin, hair, and nails look much smoother and shinier.

Before we get to the specific tips for setting yourself up for success, let's take a brief look at why some people fail with making changes to their lifestyle, including beginning to fast. Weight and health problems might result from spontaneous, unhealthy habits. From going to bed too late at night and not having enough time to prepare a healthy breakfast to spending your lunch break working only to grab a quick hamburger on the way home, you trip on the little things that snowball into major health problems.

The first step toward succeeding with fasting is to recognize those behaviors that result in sleep deprivation, delaying meals, and overeating. When you're too tired and too hungry, it's almost impossible to resist a candy bar or a heavily sweetened cup of coffee. While fasting keeps your blood sugar to a healthy minimum to prevent its spike, irregular eating does the opposite. When you avoid meals due to stress and hurry, your blood sugar levels drop below a healthy minimum. You start to feel fatigued and fear you'll get sick from hunger. The appetite you are feeling drives you to eat the first thing that comes to mind. Most often, it's not the healthiest meal. Instead, you have a sugary snack or beverage. After eating an unhealthy meal, your blood sugar spikes again, causing even more appetite. As your blood sugar yo-yos throughout the day, so does your weight in the long run. Fasting is about maintaining a balance and learning to be thoughtful of your body's needs. From this stem the following recommendations for successful fasting:

#1: Believe in Natural Healing Ability

No matter your menopausal status and age, your body has the potential to heal. The studies we talked about earlier show this. The laws of nature and biology apply to you as well. Believe that you're capable of healing and improvement.

#2: Be Patient

No matter your occupation and lifestyle, it can be too hard to go through the day without eating, especially if you need a meal before taking prescribed therapy or if other conditions demand frequent meals and snacks. For starters, introduce nighttime fasting between dinner and breakfast. Have dinner no later than 9 p.m., and breakfast no sooner than 9 a.m. You'll have achieved a week or two of 12-hour fasting easily without disrupting your daily routine.

#3: Power Up With Protein

You'll feel fuller during your fasting hours if your diet is richer in protein. Increase healthy meats, dairy, and beans, while preferably reducing carbs to a minimum. Protein breaks down much slower during the day and will keep you energized evenly throughout the day.

#4: Don't Starve Yourself!

Intermittent fasting isn't all about calorie restriction. You lose weight by speeding up your metabolism and limiting your food intake by eating only during certain hours. You still eat enough calories to maintain the fasting regimen of your choice, and you're not snacking when you're not supposed to. You eat much fewer calories than you used to because you're being mindful of your eating choices and patterns. For starters, keep your meals similar to what they used to be but on the healthier side. Just make sure to eat within your selected feeding time.

#5: Choose Strength Exercises

Although cardio is said to be most effective for weight loss, this isn't necessarily true across the board. Strength exercises are a better option for burning fat more efficiently and building muscle tissue. That's not to say that you need to buff up in your 50s if you don't want to. Strength exercises "turn your fat into muscle" in a way. The energy in fat deposits gets released to heal microtears in muscle tissue created during strength training. Muscle tissues grow as a result, while fat deposits reduce. Strength training helps even more with preventing muscle mass loss, so don't dismiss it!

#6: Get Hydrated

Make sure to have a minimum of eight daily glasses of water, and always keep a bottle of clear water by your side. Hydration helps increase the feeling of satiety, while electrolytes help cope with fatigue, headaches, and muscle pain.

HOW TO INCORPORATE INTERMITTENT FASTING INTO YOUR LIFESTYLE AND ROUTINES

Now that you know how to succeed with fasting, let's discuss establishing a routine that will work for you. If you want to make fasting a lasting habit, it's necessary to integrate it into your daily routine. Aside from choosing optimal fasting and eating times, you can use these strategies to ensure and track your progress:

#1: Measure and Track Progress

Keep your habits in check by measuring how long you can go without food and what food quantities fit you best. If you can't fully adhere to your fasting schedule, perhaps you need to increase your meal size or have more protein.

#2: Control Carb Intake

Although dietary restrictions and changes aren't a must to succeed with fasting, reducing carbs in your diet is helpful. It can induce ketosis and speed up weight loss if you substitute the same calories with protein.

#3: Plan Meals in Advance

Planning and cooking in advance ensure enough food for the whole day and prevent delaying eating until you're too hungry to make healthy choices.

2

WILL FASTING BENEFIT YOU?

Now, let's talk more about the benefits of intermittent fasting on your health and weight loss. As you learned by now, intermittent fasting affects weight loss both directly and indirectly. Directly, you lose weight as your body burns fat faster and switches between two different metabolic pathways. Aside from that, fasting benefits your overall health in many indirect ways. Here are some of them (Mackenthun, 2021):

#1: HELPS PREVENT AND IMPROVE ILLNESSES

If you've been coping with diabetes, cardiovascular disease, Parkinson's, Alzheimer's, or neurological disorders, fasting can be a great way to support your medical treatment and boost recovery. Studies have shown that people who coped with numerous chronic illnesses improved their lab results after a certain time spent fasting.

#2: CELLULAR REGENERATION

In the first chapter, you learned that your cells suffer constant damage. A part of it is normal in each cell's life cycle. As cells age and mature, they get damaged and eventually die off. They're replaced by new, healthy cells that build tissues (Mattson, 2017). However, there's a certain amount of cellular damage that occurs due to unhealthy eating, stress and exhaustion, chemicals in food and the environment, and other harmful influences. All of those damaging factors hurt your health on a cellular level. Over time, and particularly due to aging, it becomes more difficult for the body to replace damaged cells with healthy ones. When that happens, your chances of chronic diseases increase. Furthermore, the existing conditions can worsen.

As described in the first chapter, your body gets rid of damaged cells more quickly, while the increased energy flow and mitochondrial growth support the growth and multiplication of healthy cells. This promotes long-term vitality and helps you stay in good health longer.

#3: PROMOTES HEALTHY APPETITE AND INTUITIVE EATING

I suppose that you don't need a lot of convincing of the fact that the way people eat today is unhealthy. A sedentary lifestyle combined with heavily processed foods and lots of refined sugars turns our diet into everything it wasn't meant to be. Our bodies were made to eat so that we get nutrients. Our ancestors had clean, organic, nutrient-dense foods at their disposal. These foods contained higher concentrations of protein, fiber, vitamins, and minerals than we have today. Although people today live longer, and civilizational progress is admirable in many ways, a lot more people suffer from chronic illnesses than they used to.

A part of the obesity, mood disorder, diabetes, and cardiovascular epidemic can be explained by the way we eat. Now, you can debate whether or not "habits of old" should be kept. Perhaps you have better living conditions than your ancestors used to have. Yet, modern eating habits are something that humans should undoubtedly question.

Before we established the three-meal workday regimen, people ate instinctively. That is, mealtimes came when people felt they were hungry. Many people today seem to be out of touch with their natural appetites, and we no longer practice what is now called "intuitive eating." In an ideal world, you'd "listen" to your body's appetite cues. Intuitive eating has been a well-researched concept and is now recommended to people who are recovering from overeating and mood disorders.

Intuitive eating resides in the concept of cultivating a more mindful relationship with food. A purposeful, self-aware approach to one's feeding means taking the time to check in and detect your biological and emotional needs.

Nearly 50% of a person's average hunger sensation can be attributed to nervousness, tiredness, and suppressed feelings. Whether due to a busy lifestyle or emotional struggles, many people fail to address how they feel with enough self-compassion and acceptance. After all, it's hard to, for example, properly cope with a loss of a loved one when you only get a couple of days off work. After that, you're expected to bounce back and be productive, which isn't at all natural for a human being. To cope, many people choose to suppress feelings. Their sense of appetite is no longer strictly biological. It becomes emotional as well, with food being used to comfort, relax, or reward yourself.

Emotional eating doesn't have to be as deep, though. A lot of the time, we're too busy for fun, more meaningful activities. Instead of going out for a walk or spending a fun evening with friends, people prepare rich meals and have them during their favorite late-night TV show. In this case, and many others, including eating while running errands, food is a reward and a way for people to find pleasure and emotional fulfillment in the absence of time for everything else.

Of course, it's possible to work around your schedule in ways to live a more fulfilling life. But, if you've spent one or more years eating to comfort or please yourself, it creates a physiological pattern that's hard to break. This is why it's so common for people who work too much to overeat in the evening. Exhausted and without time left to spend outside, people can start to feel like eating is the only pleasure they can afford.

While you can change your daily habits and become more active, you can be left with emotional hunger that simply results from habit. Yet, this is far from healthy eating.

Studies showed that lab rats that ate spontaneously and specifically when they felt biological appetite were much healthier compared to those who ate on a trained schedule. Rats that ate on instinct were better adapted and physically and cognitively more advanced than those who weren't eating instinctively (Mattson, 2017).

As some studies showed, people who allow their bodies to be in a food-deprived state for a moderate amount of time, between 16 and 48 hours, and alter their eating patterns, enjoy better health. They also had lower chronic disease rates (Parkinson's, Alzheimer's, cancer, neurological, metabolic, and cardiovascular). To reap these benefits, it is necessary to limit your intake to an eight-hour feeding window. Reducing feeding times to eight hours or less is confirmed to trigger autophagy and spark the previously mentioned cellular regeneration.

#4: IMPROVES INSULIN RESISTANCE

Have you ever wondered what causes insulin resistance? Insulin resistance is considered to be one of the major contributors to developing type 2 diabetes. What you perhaps didn't know was that insulin resistance happens once your body starts to resist insulin. This means that your cells and tissues no longer metabolize this substance. Insulin resistance can occur in case your pancreas doesn't produce enough of it. But it can also happen due to insulin overproduction.

Unhealthy eating is said to contribute to insulin resistance because your body can no longer recognize whether you're full or hungry. A diet oversaturated with sugars and carbs causes your pancreas to excrete excess amounts of insulin, and your cells start rejecting it as a result. A vicious cycle in your body is triggered, as your cells don't get enough energy while the excess energy from blood sugar is stored within your fat cells.

When this state lasts a long time, it contributes to developing type 2 diabetes. Not only is type 2 diabetes on the rise but recovering from it is made difficult since the modern lifestyle and an abundance of unhealthy food choices make it more difficult to establish healthy habits. Aside from taking your prescribed treatment, recovery from type 2 diabetes also depends on retraining your body to produce and metabolize insulin correctly.

You see, insulin isn't an enemy to your body or health. It's not a harmful chemical that you should hate or fight against. When your body produces insulin in proportion to the food you eat, it's easy to metabolize. The amount of insulin in your blood is just enough. However, the mechanism that regulates insulin, as it turns out, is very fragile. It can be so easily thrown out of balance by irregular eating, unhealthy food, and a high-stress sedentary lifestyle. Not only is insulin resistance easy to trigger, but it also takes time to get your body on track.

This is one of the main reasons why doctors now prescribe fasting as one of the most effective lifestyle changes to support recovery from insulin resistance and type 2 diabetes. Intermittent fasting, as you recall, limits your feeding time. It "puts a cap" on the amount of insulin your body produces. When you're not eating, the production of insulin drops to a minimum, so there's no excess of it to increase weight gain and worsen type 2 diabetes. During the time you're not eating, your body can gradually recover the balance it needs for healthy functioning. Your pancreas gets "trained" regarding the amount of insulin it needs to produce while your cells gradually start to take in and metabolize insulin. The reason for this is that your cells no longer have to "protect" themselves against too much insulin. This improves your insulin sensitivity and makes your body able to produce and metabolize the exact amounts of it needed to create energy.

Aside from improving type 2 diabetes, changes that happen as a result of healing insulin resistance also affect your energy levels and mood. Insulin resistance doesn't only cause you to gain weight. It makes you sluggish and tired because all of your cells and tissues are starving for energy. As they close off to insulin as a way of protecting themselves, they're not getting the nutrition they need. This is why it's often said that you can be both obese and starving in the sense that, while your fat cells grow, your tissues and organs are thoroughly energy deprived. The sluggishness and cognitive decline that you might be facing, including imbalanced mood and lack of concentration, could be easily caused by insulin resistance.

#5: IMPROVES BETA CELL FUNCTIONING

Studies have also proven that fasting helps improve the functioning of your beta cells. Fasting was found to stimulate substances like NEUROG3 and PSMD9, which improve the health of your pancreas and help regain healthy insulin sensitivity.

On the topic of regaining the balance in your body, it's important to understand what beta cells are and their role in weight loss and preventing insulin resistance. With hyperglycemia, these cells begin to die out, and your body no longer produces enough glucose. This worsens diabetes and makes your recovery more difficult.

Fasting was found to stimulate the autophagy flux, which promotes the growth and development of beta cells.

#6: ACTIVATES THE AUTOPHAGY-LYSOSOME PATHWAY

Aside from improving the performance of your pancreas, promoting better cell regeneration, and inducing weight loss, fasting also triggers the Autophagy-Lysosome Pathway. In simple terms, this metabolic pathway is the mechanism behind your body's ability to break down damaged cells and tissues and further use the energy to make itself better, healthier, and stronger. Call it self-recycling, if you will, as autophagy helps prevent the build-up of diseased and damaged cells in your body. It sparks a physiological process during which those cells are broken down into energy, and that same energy is henceforth used for cell regeneration. Isn't that amazing?

Even better, studies have verified this. Researchers found that fasting stimulates the production of proteins that regulate the autophagy mechanisms in your pancreas. This was proven by measuring the lab tests of experimental mice who've been on a fasting regimen to measure the effects on their body and whether or not fasting will induce autophagy (Liu, et. al., 2017).

#7: REDUCES TRIACYLGLYCEROL LEVELS IN YOUR LIVER AND PANCREAS

Numerous studies showed that fasting helps lower triacylglycerol levels in your liver. This was proven by numerous tests done on rats that showed declining levels of triacylglycerol while increasing the healthy beta cells. Altogether, this helps prevent insulin resistance.

#8: PROMOTES LONGEVITY

Experimental rats and mice that were used in studies that measured the effects of intermittent fasting had longer life spans compared to the control group of subjects. While testing this assumption on humans would require studies too long to be attainable so soon into the implementation of this lifestyle, it's reasonable to assume that a well-thought-out fasting regimen would prolong one's life beyond what it would be without fasting.

There are numerous potential explanations behind the theory that fasting promotes longevity. A part of it can be attributed to the fact that fasting reduces cardiovascular disease, diabetes, obesity, and other chronic illnesses that are dubbed the leading causes of death. If you choose to fast, whether for weight loss or health, your chances of succumbing to some of the most life-threatening illnesses will notably decrease (Ganesan et al., 2018).

#9: PREVENTS TUMOR GROWTH

Functional autophagy was found to slow down tumor growth. How? It's simple. After your body burns through excess fatty deposits, it begins metabolizing diseased cells. Of course, tumor and cancer cells are among the cells that the body starts to naturally break down. Yet, autophagy can't still be considered the hallmark of healing. As it turns out, there's a downside to this process, and it is in the activation of biological processes that promote tumor growth. This is why your doctor will likely recommend maintaining an optimal weight past desired weight loss. After your body breaks down its excess fat and unhealthy cells, autophagy may start to affect healthy cells. To keep your autophagy functional, it's recommended to fast at longer intervals yet fewer times throughout the year. Experts recommend alternating a month or two of stricter intermittent fasting with a regular eating schedule to prevent damage to healthy tissues and organs.

#10: PROMOTES SHORT-TERM WEIGHT LOSS

Losing a visible amount of weight within a short period perhaps looks like a distant fantasy. Maybe you were told that the only healthy weight loss is slow. Of course, a well-meaning dietician will tell you this to prevent extreme calorie restriction. Fad diets reside on the false assumption that the fewer calories you eat, the greater weight loss you experience.

While this isn't true for starvation diets, studies found that people were able to drop significant amounts of weight regardless of whether they had normal weight or they were overweight or obese (Ganesan et al., 2018).

Rapid yet healthy weight loss often results from a combination of different influences. Not only does your body burn fat faster as a result of ketosis, but better general health makes you more energized and active. You start to burn even more calories, now with being more outgoing. Aside from that, fasting helps you regain control over your appetite and eating. With your insulin production being optimal, you no longer feel the need to eat beyond your nutritional needs. However, these studies also showed that longer fasting periods were more efficient in inducing the mentioned health benefits. The results applied regardless of whether or not the study participants reduced calorie intake.

However, it's important to remember that not everyone reacts the same to fasting. While some study participants felt like their appetite dropped, others got hungrier as a result of restricted eating.

As you can see, there are more than enough reasons for you to try and persist with fasting, no matter how challenging it may look. Remember, if you plan your fasting regimen well and consider those times of day when you're most tired, as well as your capacity to shop and prepare foods, you will succeed.

I can't say how long exactly it will take for you to start noticing health and weight loss benefits. Some people experience their first results within a week, while others struggle for months to get into a routine that works for them. With that in mind, here are a couple of additional considerations to boost the benefits of fasting:

Consult your doctor. At the time of writing this book, intermittent fasting has become accepted among physicians. After all, doctors tend to acknowledge scientific findings. However, your doctor may advise caution or recommend a gradual fasting regimen to secure your well-being throughout. With so many different fasting regimens to choose from, you should get expert advice on the feeding times that will work best for you. Your doctor will account for your lifestyle and how active you are, as well as your health history and current treatments. If you're taking medication several times throughout the day, your doctor might recommend a wider feeding window so that you can take your medication before or after a meal.

Get local advice. My experience with intermittent fasting diet plans shows that every community has its specific culinary culture. Your geographic background may determine the foods at your disposal and looking online for a diet plan may not be as practical as needed for success. For this reason, the recipes given in this book are based on the most widespread foods that you can find in your nearest grocery store, and they're also quick and easy to make. Yet, to keep up the lifestyle in the long run, you'll need to discover which common meals fit the best. Don't burden yourself with trying to keep up some innovative, exotic, or expensive meal plan. Instead, go for the simplest healthy options, and you won't find it hard.

Planning trumps trying. Sadly, I have seen people give up on fasting as the regimen was seemingly too hard to attain. The main reasons were the lack of time to shop and pre-make meals, hence lacking healthy options throughout the feeding window. To avoid this, get your groceries and plan for time to cook and eat at least a week ahead. This will give you enough time to prepare and reduce the chance of skipping meals during your designated time, only to break your fast later in the day.

3

INTERMITTENT FASTING FOR WOMEN OVER 50

In the first chapter, you learned more about why it's so hard to lose weight after 50. There are numerous factors affecting your metabolism. Hormonal changes, loss of muscle mass, appetite changes, and altered sleep patterns can all diminish your capacity to slim down. You also learned why fasting is such a great way to instill a permanent change into your lifestyle. Fasting doesn't only boost your metabolism; it helps you become more energized and uplifted, with less brain fog and better concentration.

You also learned that, consequently, fasting can improve your health on a cellular level. You learned that fasting helps your cells regenerate, and it also helps prevent the same chronic illnesses that are to blame for the vast majority of negative outcomes and loss of life.

Intermittent fasting has been proven effective for people of both genders and all age groups, which makes it a great option for women over 50 who are looking for a healthy life change.

Yet, if implementing changes was so easy, you wouldn't need this book. You'd simply look up the most popular fasting regimens and decide which feeding times work best for you. It's the plurality of options for fasting that imposes the need to better understand what's going on inside your body, how it works amid this transformative life stage, and how you can work together with the biological mechanisms in your body to foster healthy changes.

HORMONAL CHANGES IN WOMEN AFTER 50

Aside from the changes that happen with aging alone, there are hormonal changes specific to women who are approaching menopause. These changes feel challenging at times as they result from a changing hormonal balance in your body. More importantly, these changes affect how you metabolize food and how your body spends and stores energy.

If your understanding of menopause has been vague, let's give it a bit more clarity. Menopause is a year after your last menstrual cycle. However, the most visible changes in your body and mood begin to show in the years before your menopause. You might start to notice that your monthly cycles are changing and that you're experiencing hot flashes. The changes leading up to menopause start approximately at the age of 45 but may appear as late as 55. After all, each woman's body is unique. During this time called perimenopause or pre-menopause, your hormones fluctuate and vary.

During the period of approaching menopause, known as perimenopause, and the menopause itself, your estrogen levels begin to fluctuate. These fluctuations are more intense and significant than those you'd experience throughout your usual monthly cycle. Estrogen production becomes rather unpredictable before it eventually drops to its minimal levels during menopause.

But, before your body settles into a new balance, your other hormones, including thyroid hormones, cortisol, serotonin, and sex hormones, will fluctuate as well. This creates uncomfortable symptoms that are typical for menopause (Galang, 2022).

While some women don't experience major symptoms of menopause, others might experience problems with sleep, hot flashes, and pain while having sex. Once the menopausal symptoms begin, women might think that they can no longer get pregnant. However, there's no certainty of that before your doctor can verify that you can no longer conceive.

Yet, these symptoms aren't limited to some of the discomforts that you might be feeling. Your metabolism undergoes numerous changes as well, and some of these changes may leave you more vulnerable to insulin resistance. Before and during menopause, your insulin sensitivity reduces. As your cells become less sensitive to insulin, they take in less of this substance to metabolize it and use it for energy.

Now, what happens when your insulin sensitivity starts to reduce? Your body begins to struggle to break down and process sugars and carbs. Once your body can no longer break down sugar the way it used to, pounds may start to pile up around your belly, waist, and thighs.

As your muscle mass reduces and the fatty deposits increase, you can start to have difficulty slimming down and getting rid of that stubborn fat. As you know by now, intermittent fasting is helpful to trigger your metabolism and induce fat burning. How?

Remember, during the time you're not eating, your body needs to rely on an alternate source of energy, given that blood glucose is at its lowest. This is a simple mechanism that works regardless of your age group.

Plainly and simply, your body needs an energy source, and when there's no blood glucose to provide that immediate supply, it must turn to expend calories from fat. But fasting helps you lose weight and improve health in more than a single way (Carb Manager, 2022):

Muscle Gain Hormones

Fasting promotes the production of human growth hormone (HGH). This hormone supports fat-burning and muscle growth. Why is this so important? It can be hard to find a diet that works for you after 50, given the lesser physical activity, muscle loss, and slower metabolism. Diets are hard to introduce at this age during the risks associated with calorie restriction.

Many physicians will prescribe a diet when they feel a woman will benefit from it, but with a lot of caution in regard to how many calories should be cut down. Eating too few calories can have the exact opposite effect: your body further slows down the metabolism to preserve energy, muscle mass is further depleted and used to obtain energy instead of fat, and naturally, your health declines as a result of energy and nutrient deficiency.

Better Portion Control

Instead of taking a risk with fad diets, you can opt in to fasting, which doesn't require you to eat significantly less to reduce weight. Yet, fasting does lead to women eating fewer calories over time. This is because fasting fosters a better, healthier relationship with food. When you limit your meals to a single feeding window, there's less chance of snacking late in the day or randomly pulling out food from the fridge when your blood sugar temporarily drops. One of the ways fasting helps you control appetite is biological, and it consists of balancing your hunger and satiety hormone. But the second way lies in fostering a more thoughtful relationship with yourself and your hunger. Knowing that your daily meals will be limited to a certain feeding window means that you'll take a closer look at what you want and should eat during that time.

When all of your meals are condensed in a short time frame, you get to review them all and figure out whether you eat too much or too little. Would you believe that many overweight women eat too little during the day and overcompensate for the loss of energy in the evening? You'll no longer do this once you start to fast. Why? You'll gain insight into how much you eat versus how much (and what) you should be eating.

Improved Insulin Sensitivity

As you get increasingly vulnerable to insulin resistance, it becomes vital that you do your best and preserve a healthy level of insulin sensitivity. Healthy insulin sensitivity allows your cells to metabolize and use insulin healthfully without leaving the excess substance to be processed into energy for fat cells. Studies showed that fasting helped a group of obese women reduce insulin levels significantly within six months (Stanton, 2021)!

Improved Mental Health

By now, you have learned that fasting and the phenomenon of autophagy that it triggers help improve the beta cells in your body. But it also helps improve mental health throughout the weight-loss period and overall. Many women struggle with their mood, self-esteem, and anxiousness as a result of weight. Going on a diet is stressful as it entails being hungry and not eating as much as you're used to, yet still spending a great deal of time and effort on shopping, food prep, and cooking. On top of that, it might take up to two or three months for a diet to produce visible results.

Add to that the effects of hormonal fluctuations and body change typical for women over 50, and you can get an idea about how mentally challenging weight loss can get. Perimenopausal and menopausal symptoms don't only include uncomfortable physical sensations. They can also cause anxiousness, severe mood swings, brain fog, fatigue, and anxiety. For some women, psychological stress is so severe that they might experience intense anxiety and depression. Luckily, studies found that fasting can even help regulate mood, and it can overall help improve your quality of life. While there were no studies that examined the impact of this lifestyle on the brain, we can deduce that fasting reduces the hormones and other substances that are to blame for mood disorders, like cortisol, while increasing those that help you feel calm and optimistic, such as serotonin, melatonin, and oxytocin.

Since the majority of knowledge and information that we have on fasting comes from general studies and those done on laboratory animals, you'll need a closer look at findings that concern women older than 50 specifically.

HOW INTERMITTENT FASTING BENEFITS WOMEN OVER 50

Women's bodies are different compared to men's and most certainly different from those of laboratory animals that were used to conduct experiments. Women process food differently and have different metabolic patterns and hormonal balance. This is why you need more knowledge on how to make fasting work for you.

Now, let's reflect on some research studies that examined the effects of eating regimens. What makes these studies important is that they focused on various aspects of women's health and weight loss with aging.

Studies found that fasting helped older women lose belly fat and decreased their risks of developing metabolic syndrome. Why is this important? As you age, you start to notice that the shape of your body is changing and that you're no longer gaining weight the same way you used to. Perhaps you didn't use to gain a lot in your arms, shoulders, and belly, yet those parts of your body now seem to get larger easily. Aside from giving your body a shape that you don't necessarily appreciate, weight gain starts to affect your mood and energy levels much more quickly.

Studies also showed that fasting affected how women's bodies produced bone tissues, leading to the conclusion that it also improved bone health. Bones tend to get more brittle with aging, and you may start to feel like you're no longer as flexible as you used to be. You might start to feel pain in your joints, back, and hips as a result. Luckily, you have a strategy at hand that can help heal those pains.

Mental health aspects showed that different fasting regimens improved overall mental well-being. Aside from alleviating pains and improving hormonal balance, women who fasted seemed to enjoy a more balanced and overall calmer, optimistic mood.

When it comes to the downsides of intermittent fasting, only one notably stands out, and it is the potential to trigger or promote the growth of tumorous cells.

If you recall from the earlier chapters, we mentioned that some studies discovered the potential for fasting to promote the growth of tumorous cells if not implemented and used correctly. To prevent this risk, it's best to ask your doctor whether or not intermittent fasting is a healthy solution for you.

Did you know that fasting can help with PCOS? Some studies showed that fasting helped women with PCOS improve metabolic and endocrine profiles. These studies showed that 75% of women who fasted for five weeks had more regular cycles compared to women with PCOS who didn't fast. Although the direct connection between PCOS hasn't been proven, intermittent fasting is proven to disrupt estrogen levels, which consequently links with PCOS.

TIPS TO STAY SLIM DURING MENOPAUSE

Now, let's talk a bit more about what you can do to increase success with intermittent fasting. You see, following general recommendations for fasting won't necessarily yield the improvements you were hoping to see. Success with fasting comes from understanding your body well and applying strategies that were shown to work specifically for women in menopause. This is important to remember as the majority of studies in this area were done either on the general population, younger people, or animals. The results of these studies won't necessarily apply to you if you don't understand how your metabolism is changing and what makes your body different. Here are a couple of useful strategies to make fasting easier and more efficient:

Understand Your Metabolism

Accept that the way you process food is now changing. A new weight gain pattern appears where your body gets fuller in your torso and shoulders and flatter in your legs and behind. While some women embrace this shape, others don't feel like wearing it if there is a way out of it:

- **Skip breakfast if possible.** Since your feeding time is limited to a certain number of hours, it's good to concentrate your meals on those hours when you need energy and nutrition the most. For example, if you work a full nine-to-five shift, you'll likely feel most exhausted toward the end of the day. In that case, have your breakfast around noon and lunch during the mid-day break. Then, have a satisfying dinner to keep you going until the next day. On the other hand, if you work in the afternoon and in the evenings, you might benefit from starting your feeding window around 2-3 p.m. and stretching it throughout the day to supply yourself with enough energy and calories. Most people have a big breakfast on instinct or by habit, even if they don't have a particularly active morning. The majority of the energy from your breakfast will then be spent on idle activities, leaving you tired and starving during the busiest time of the day. This isn't good, wouldn't you agree? Unless your lifestyle and occupation dictate a particularly busy morning, perhaps it wouldn't be bad to just start your day with a simple cup of black coffee.

- **Remember that ketosis is optional.** More time-restricted eating will help you slip into ketosis but think about whether or not you want or need it. There are some conditions, rare diseases, and autoimmune diseases. Although studies generally agree that ketosis may help manage some symptoms of difficult illnesses, the reduction in micronutrients and fiber is said to harm digestion, which could create other difficult symptoms. If you're not sure that ketosis is good for you, or you were advised against keto by your physician, consider expanding your food choices with only the healthiest carbs. At the same time, keep the carbs to a minimum to support the natural healing processes that are going to unfold with fasting.

- **Drink black coffee and tea.** Even if you wish to have a cup of coffee or tea outside your eating times, you can do so without breaking your fast. What technically breaks fast is insulin, and if the beverages you take don't stimulate your insulin production, you'll be fine.

- **Drink lemon water to suppress appetite.** If you struggle to keep away from food during your periods of fasting, try lemon water. It is said that this beverage helps better control appetite. Plus, you'll get some more hydration, which is always a good thing.

- **Start from a 12-hour fast, and increase gradually to 14,15, and eventually 16 hours of fasting.** The half-day fast is as close to regular eating as possible. However, it still entails that you're mindful of your calorie intake and food choices. Your twelve-hour fast may sound easy but think about limiting your meals to a window between 8 a.m. and 8 p.m., for example. This means that you can't have dinner past 8 p.m., even if you don't have the time to eat sooner. You'll be skipping a meal and saying 'no' to late-night snacks, which is still a major adjustment from your previous habits. Once you get used to eating only during the designated time and eating clean, healthy foods, you can start shortening your eating times and fasting longer.

- **Practice one day of 500-calorie restriction for two days a month.** Some experts recommend occasionally doing a more rigorous fast to jump-start your metabolism, particularly if you're advised against long-term intermittent fasting by your physician. Such intense breaks from food may not feel good, but they benefit your body and spark all of those healing processes that may have slowed down.

If you find it hard to fast every day, you can practice the so-called "Eat-stop-eat" fast every other day. This means that you'll fast for 24 hours at least once a week. This, however, doesn't mean that you have to go an entire day without food. You can begin your fast after dinner and then fast until tomorrow night, when you'll have dinner again.

Don't Deprive Yourself of Pleasure and Socializing

Intermittent fasting shouldn't keep you from enjoying your life to the fullest. You shouldn't obsess about eating and refuse to meet with friends and family simply because they'll serve food at an inconvenient time, or you'll find it difficult not to eat all those delicious pies, pizzas, pasta, and pastries.

Fasting, and even going on keto, doesn't mean that you need to give up on those rich family meals or only order lean dishes when going out with your friends. Some experts on fasting recommend going on a stricter fast a day or two before you plan on going out, taking a trip, or attending an event where you'll want to treat yourself with some "guilty pleasures."

Write Down Your Food Intake

It's easy to spontaneously snack and drink sugary beverages throughout the day and not even realize it. We tend to forget how many calories certain foods and beverages contain simply because they don't look "lean." Examples of this would be fruit salads, nut butter, whole nuts and seeds, and other snacks. But, if you look closer, you'll realize that a bag of nuts or a cup of sweetened coffee with cream and syrup easily contains the same number of calories as a rich portion of a home-cooked meal. Write down everything you eat and check how many calories your food contains to avoid eating more than your burn. Regardless of fasting, eating more calories than you spend could still result in weight gain! Do this for only a couple days, and you'll start to develop an eating intuition and the right perspective of the calories you're eating. You'll no longer have to write things down because you'll have a pretty good idea of how much you're eating.

As you can see, there are plenty of things that you can do to improve your health and weight. You might not be in control of the aging process, which dictates how your body changes, but you certainly are able to control all other aspects of your diet and lifestyle that affect how these changes will unfold and how they will affect you. Whenever you start to feel powerless in the face of aging and illness, keep in mind that you're always in control of the following:

- **Your relationship with food.** Remember that your eating decisions produce instant and severe consequences for your health. You hold the power to turn your back on toxic chemicals, sweeteners, and processed sugars found in packaged foods.

- **Physical activity.** You have a choice whether to stay up late and watch TV or go to bed earlier so that you have more time and energy for a quick jog or even a mindful walk in the fresh air. Prioritizing health over entertainment may not feel 'cool,' but it will help gain mental clarity and willpower to engage in making healthy eating choices.
- **Decisions and learning.** Instead of making spontaneous decisions about what to eat, make educated ones. Learn more about how many calories you need each day and what foods will give you the exact macronutrient ratio you're looking for. It might look weird to read about the nutritional values of each food you eat, but the positive effects of it will snowball into better physical and mental health.

4

MINDSET TO PREPARE FOR FASTING

Great job! You're almost halfway through this book, and you already know the many secrets to succeed with intermittent fasting. Now, it's time to address one of the most important success principles, and that is having the right mindset. Knowing how to think about fasting and your diet and learning how to control hunger impulses when your strength is put to the test helps you stay strong along the way.

To start on a positive note, remember that fasting is very easy and affordable. Restraining yourself from eating outside the feeding time only means that you'll spend less money on snacks and less time cooking and prepping food. Soon, you'll notice that your grocery costs are reducing, and the amount of free time is increasing. Adding a slimmer figure to the list of amazing effects that fasting will have on your life will only empower you to push further.

AWAKEN YOUR FOOD CONSCIOUSNESS

The very fact that you're transitioning from a lifestyle of habitual eating to that of more mindful, controlled eating is a major turning point in a woman's life. How do we go from eating whatever we want and whenever we want while staying slim to struggling to drop a pound a month?

A part of the answer to this question lies in biology and the changes that happen in your body as you mature. Yet, the bigger influences are those of how we shift our mindset from taking good care of our bodies to prioritizing everything else over our health and well-being. Look back at your time in high school. You not only enjoyed the invigorating energy of youth, but your well-being was much more controlled and looked after. Your health was literally someone else's responsibility, whether your family, school, or the health system. By the time you started working and/or got to college, you still had plenty of free time to take care of yourself. You had hours to rest whenever you needed, and you could virtually take an entire afternoon for some careful grocery shopping.

All of this changes with adulthood for both men and women. Although health issues remain consistent regardless of gender, particularly those that concern diet and lifestyle, there are some habits that are more typical for women than they are for men. If you raised children, you know how quickly women's physiological needs drop to the very bottom of the priority list. Both men and women tend to neglect healthy eating, sleeping, and physical activity when starting families. This is justified to a degree, but when there's no longer an immediate need for it, you should start getting back to your healthy habits and start thinking more about your health.

If raising a family wasn't the thing that got you to knock yourself down the priority list, it could have been your career and other responsibilities. Either way, adulthood makes it terribly difficult for both men and women to take good care of themselves. Not only eating but also sleeping and exercising becomes a privilege for those with plenty of time to spare, or at least it appears to be the case. Yet, declining health can often make you wonder if your sacrifice was worth it. Can you truly enjoy everything you achieved in life when you're suffering from health issues and hemorrhaging money on medical bills? It's common for that priority scale to tip on the side of your own well-being around the time you face life-turning health problems. If that hasn't happened yet, it's time to start thinking about yourself!

The first major mindset change to adopt is the one from neglecting your needs to taking good care of your nutrition, health, and well-being (Fung, 2019).

Food Exposure

Our bodies have adapted to fasting. It is entirely natural for the human body to go a longer number of hours without food. Yet, the majority of the struggle you experience is mental. Humans are wired to notice food, and its very presence triggers biological responses. Don't blame your body! Your body is a miracle of millions of years of evolution, out of which food has never been as abundant in the Western world as it has been for the last 100 years. Your primal mind was designed during the time when food was seen to be eaten. There wasn't a lot of it, and even if there was, you had to eat in a hurry before a wild animal got you. It's hard to control that primitive mechanism that triggers appetite because it was made strong and resilient.

Let's briefly address the presence of food around you. Whether or not you're hungry at the moment, you likely have more food at your disposal than needed. You likely own enough snacks, way beyond needed for staying healthy. Have you ever wondered how much of your hunger is justified and how much of it is triggered by food exposure?

Start thinking more about your perception of food and thought patterns associated with eating. Grab a piece of paper and a pen and write down your memories of walking the streets and seeing all the restaurants, food stands, and flyers. Aren't they all appetizing? Write down what the experience feels like and how often you ate simply because you discovered a new, interesting stand or dinner, regardless of whether or not you were hungry.

Habitual Eating

Do you eat simply because it's lunchtime? Or you're grabbing a quick snack before your meeting because you don't want your stomach to growl. Start unpacking your thoughts regarding eating times.

Begin thinking about all the times you eat out of boredom or for emotional purposes rather than purely biological. Granted, mindful eating embraces extracting fulfillment from food, but it focuses more on how the food benefits your body and health rather than using food to obtain the kind of fulfillment that we should be getting from fun activities, creative work, and relationships.

Unconscious Eating

How does one eat unconsciously? Do you fall out of consciousness and then get up to eat before you wake up? Not really. Unconscious eating actually means eating without being aware that you're eating. You're stretching at home, taking a break from working on your laptop, and you're randomly spilling a glass of juice down your throat with a handful of peanuts. You barely think of it and even eat your next regular meal without any recollection of having eaten an entire meal before, yet you have. A handful of nuts with a glass of a sugary beverage can have up to 600 calories, which equates to eating a small steak with a side dish. Yet, it's nowhere near as satiating, and the calories from the said meal are injected into your fat cells faster than you know.

Tracking your eating, even before you start fasting, is essential to end unconscious eating. Here's a challenge: For a single day, don't eat anything without writing it down. Sit down at the end of the day and calculate how many calories, as well as carbs, your spontaneous snacks contained. You can easily conclude that you had well over 1,000 calories without even knowing!

This simple exercise is often enough to help women stop unconscious eating, as it makes you more aware of how sporadic bites can cause weight gain over time.

After you've calculated the number of calories that you eat unconsciously, think about the following: You only need 20 extra calories per day to gain weight long-term.

Eating Out of Humility

Do you find yourself thinking it's ungrateful or arrogant to refuse food or not finish your meal because so many people starve? If so, start thinking more helpful thoughts. If you don't feel like finishing a meal, then simply don't. You can donate leftovers or freeze them for a later time when you'll need a quick meal without enough time to cook.

Avoiding Wasting Food

Eating more than you need simply to throw away food is a common trap for women trying to slim down. When was the last time you cooked a dish that you didn't plan on making simply because your fridge was filled with food that was about to expire? Avoid doing this moving forward, and instead of throwing away food, consider donating or giving it away to friends and family.

Eating in Advance

I bet most women can relate to eating ahead of time. When you expect to have a busy or emotionally excruciating day, you may want to prepare yourself both physically and mentally by eating a lot in advance. This is a mistake that can easily cause overeating. Instead, measure your portion based on the recommended calorie intake and macronutrient ratio. When you focus on the quantities you're eating rather than the composition of your meal, it's more likely that you'll make unhealthy choices. When you put more thought into what your meal will look like, you'll find that, for example, adding a slice or two of meat to your meal will make it a lot more satiating without the need to increase its carb portion.

Social Eating

How many meals so far have you had simply because you were offered one? It's often hard to decline hospitality, even when the foods prepared aren't healthy or good for you. Perhaps you're not even that hungry, but you'll still accept your friend's offer to order a pizza because you want the two of you to have more fun. Food is often used to "set the tone" for get-togethers, as it evokes warm feelings of abundance and togetherness. It's okay to step away from this arrangement if it compromises your health or simply enjoy the ambiance without eating outside your eating window.

Being overly focused on eating is sometimes a part of a woman's lifestyle. As women age, they start to pay more attention to cooking because they have more time to fill and to please their loved ones. Nothing wrong with that, except that you don't necessarily have to be the one to eat. Take a closer look at whether you're obsessing with food, from thinking too much about getting groceries to arranging your entire schedule around mealtimes.

FASTING MINDSET CHANGES TO ADOPT

For many women, a lifestyle that revolves too much around eating starts when they start their own families. Small children and youth do need regular family meals, and for a good number of years, parents' lifestyles are heavily dictated by their children's daily regimens. This is only justified to the degree to which it's necessary. If you wish to maintain a steady mealtime in your home, feel free to do so. But start to view your diet separately from everyone else's. It's alright to eat a bit earlier or a bit later than everyone else if your health and shape are in question.

To get there, it's necessary to set yourself up for success by cultivating a healthy fasting mindset. This includes the awareness of the following:

#1: Stay Hydrated

Water isn't just an empty liquid. It plays a huge role in replenishing your body with minerals and electrolytes. It can be considered nutrition in a way, but in such a form that doesn't break your fast, autophagy, or ketosis with insulin increases. Instead, drinking water helps manage your appetite while you're not eating. Drinking water, herbal teas, and coffee temporarily tricks your body into thinking that your stomach is full. This helps you cope with your appetite until the time comes for you to eat again.

#2: Keep Yourself From Thinking About Eating

Excluding unhealthy sugars and carbs from your diet will undoubtedly cause some withdrawal in the first week of your fasting routine. Once you get the hang of fasting, you'll no longer struggle with hunger outside the eating window. But, during the initial stages, you'll just have to push through the faux hunger, which might get pretty intense. One way to cope is to keep track of your eating so that you can be certain that the appetite you're feeling isn't a real one. Knowing that you ate as much food as needed to function healthfully throughout the day helps you convince yourself that you're indeed coping with a false appetite. An even better way to cope is to find ways to distract yourself from thinking about food overall. What's typical for people who struggle with weight is that they occupy themselves with food a lot. If food is a major factor in your life, and you spend a lot of time thinking about what you'll eat, how you'll cook it, and what you need to get, it means that a mindset shift is in order. Just thinking about food can cause hunger, whether or not you need to eat.

Learning how to distract yourself from thinking about food simultaneously helps heal from all of those unconscious behaviors that caused you to eat too many calories in the first place. Ask yourself, "Why am I thinking about food so much?" What most people discover is that food itself is a distraction from tiredness and boredom, sometimes both at once. It takes genuine effort to plan a fulfilling lifestyle. If you wish to transform your life, plan for activities ahead of time. Plan out your day so that it's filled with fun, enjoyable activities that will keep you from thinking about food. Take evening walks, read a book, or call a friend instead of sitting down to snack and watch TV.

#3: Ride the Hunger Waves

A good part of managing hunger is realizing that it's not dangerous. Most people have an instinct to fear hunger and avoid it, even though it really can't harm them. Your sensation of hunger is a product of your hunger hormone. Ignore it, and it's bound to go away as the chemical "wears off." While genuine, biological hunger increases over time to the point of feeling sick unless you eat; the so-called "hormonal" or "chemical" hunger comes and goes. During the initial stages of your fast, you may experience these waves of hunger. Acknowledge how you feel, but also recognize that the sensation is harmless and is by no means a reason to break your fast.

#4: Be Sure You Should Be Fasting

Although fasting is generally thought of as healthy, there are some categories of people who shouldn't fast. There are some instances when fasting could cause harmful side effects. Don't start fasting unless your clinician has explicitly approved it regarding your unique health history and lab results. These categories of women are typically advised against fasting:

- **Pregnant women.** If you're pregnant or you're breastfeeding your infant, you need a slight daily calorie increase and enough sugar in your diet to supply both your and the baby's nutrition. If you fast, you might risk your blood sugar dropping too low or not providing yourself and the baby enough macronutrients for healthy growth and development.

- **Trying to conceive.** Women who are trying to conceive shouldn't put their bodies through additional strain. Fasting can ignite physiological and biochemical processes that might get in the way of the regular menstrual cycle. In this case, fasting could affect fertility. Women who wish to control their weight and keep blood sugar in check while trying to get pregnant should ask their clinician for the best nutrition options. They might be better off with a balanced, low-carb diet that includes a wider variety of foods while keeping the calories within a healthy frame.

- **Children.** Growing kiddos need their carbs and fats in healthy amounts. Granted, children shouldn't eat otherwise unhealthy foods either, as obesity has become an epidemic among children as well. However, children should have a versatile, well-balanced diet with timely meals that meet all of their nutritional needs.

- **Women with low blood sugar.** Given that fasting primarily aims to lower blood sugar, women who are taking medication for low blood sugar should avoid it. If you start fasting against your clinician's advice, you're increasing your risk of hypoglycemia.

- **Women with nutrition deficiency.** There are numerous reasons why a woman would have an increased need for healthy nutrients. Those who are malnourished, have a history of eating disorders, or are vulnerable to eating disorder tendencies should avoid fasting. Given that it's restrictive, fasting could trigger symptoms in those who have or are recovering from eating disorders.

#5: Distract Yourself With Fun Activities

Unless your appetite is biological, there's no good reason to eat. If you've followed the advice given in this book so far, you know how to tell the difference between emotional and biological appetite. Instead of eating to cope with boredom or a bad mood, cheer yourself up with some music, a nice book, or outdoor activity.

#6: Embrace Failure and Keep Going

One of the major reasons why women, as well as men, give up helpful changes is failure. The minute we fail, we start to think that the positive change we're trying to introduce isn't for us. If you have tried fasting before and have broken your fast the very first night, you might think that you might not be able to keep it up. However, failure is an important part of learning through trial and error. Look at the reasons why fasting, or any other positive life change, didn't work for you, and learn from it.

#7: Assume Control and Believe In Your Power

Women are stripped of a sense of personal power from childhood. Both girls and boys, each in their unique way, are made to feel powerless as children and then made to build unhealthy coping mechanisms. Our male counterparts may rely too much on physical strength, aggression, and emotional suppression to regain a sense of control. We ladies, on the other hand, are too often encouraged to convey powerlessness as means to get help, compassion, and empathy.

While both genders face their unique challenges, it's common for women to have less confidence in their ability to eat less. If you've often caught yourself fearing that you'll faint from hunger or that less eating will affect your job performance, you're not alone! The solution is to realize that everything you do is a result of your choices. If you set out to do good work, you'll do so even if you didn't have that huge dinner the night before. You'll go through half of the day on an empty stomach, and chances are that you won't get sick. The more you test and challenge yourself, the more you'll believe in your strengths and abilities.

#8: Embrace the Challenges of Detoxing

Your self-image reflects what you think about your abilities, and in return, that mindset affects the outcomes of your actions. More importantly, it affects the actions that you choose to take. As we're naturally taught to avoid negative consequences, the initial temporary discomfort brought on by fasting can make you think that you won't have enough strength to pull through.

Instead of giving up, identify how you can make things easier on yourself. Think about the times when you tend to face the biggest challenges and the best ways to cope with them. For example, if you start craving sweets and you feel sluggish, you need a better way to resolve this situation instead of eating. Go out and have fun, whether it's engaging in a creative project or going outside for some fresh air.

#9: Team Up With Supporters

Joining groups and communities devoted to fasting will help make the transition easier. You'll face similar challenges as your friends and fasting peers, and that way, you'll realize you're not alone. Plus, having someone to keep you company will make the journey more fun. Fun and friends tend to stimulate healthy hormones like oxytocin and endorphins, all of which contribute to less hunger and a greater feeling of ease and relaxation.

#10: Celebrate Your Progress

It took years to gain excess weight. In the same way it took time to gain weight, losing it might take even longer. You shouldn't be so hard on yourself if you're struggling, but instead, celebrate the choice you made. Reflect on everything you learned, and praise yourself for deciding to make smarter, healthier choices. You might not have hit your target with the number of pounds you wanted to lose. But you haven't eaten sugar in days, and stress-eating is ancient history. All of these changes will help you live a longer, more fulfilling life, regardless of how much you weigh. Write down all of your achievements and turn to your list if your confidence is ever shaken.

The crucial part of changing your mindset with intermittent fasting is realizing that you're shifting from using food for the wrong purposes to using it to nourish and build your body. Whenever you encounter a challenge, reflect on the importance of and the size of the change you're making. Forgive yourself for mistakes made, and simply pick up where you left off.

5

LIFESTYLE VERSUS DIET

Did you start reading this book thinking that intermittent fasting is a diet? If so, you wouldn't be the first to make that mistake. Most people confuse fasting for a form of dieting because the lifestyle itself mostly relies on changing your eating habits. Yet, as you're about to learn, fasting has more profound meaning and more significant aspects that exceed its dietary effects.

While adhering to intermittent fasting principles will reflect on your diet the most, you'll learn how to make significant changes that will benefit your health long-term.

WHY DON'T DIETS WORK?

So, what's the core problem with diets, and why don't they seem to work? Despite the growing weight loss industry, obesity seems to remain a prevalent disease among children and adults in the United States, and it is considered to be one of the leading causes of life-threatening illnesses.

To unwrap all of the reasons why diets don't work and arguably to discover how you can find an easy way to eat that does work, we first need to make a brief detour to biological mechanisms that govern our nutrition. At the very core, food is a tool for the human body to obtain energy. Energy is a way for your body to function and for each of your organs to do its purpose. As such, diets can neither be good nor bad per se, but instead, how you use them can have a beneficial or detrimental effect on your body. If nutrition was only about "calories in, calories out," our lives would be so much easier! But your food is more than that. Calories alone don't determine the effect of food on your body, but rather the size and composition of your meal.

All nutrients that you take consist of macronutrients and micronutrients. Macronutrients include fat, protein, and carbohydrates. Micronutrients include vitamins, minerals, and other beneficial substances that are found in different amounts in different foods. When you eat your meal, your combined foods all get broken down and digested, and their nutrients are used to fuel biological processes and build tissues and organs. Where does the problem occur? Different nutrients need different metabolic processes to be broken down and used for energy. Ideally, these processes would be somewhat equally active in your body (you already know that metabolic shifts are beneficial for health and weight loss). The problem is when, due to the way you eat, one metabolic pathway is more active than the other ones, yet you still eat food containing different macronutrients. That way, only a portion of what you eat does the job of energizing and building the body, while the rest is either ejected from the body or stored in fat. If you eat carb-saturated foods for too long, your metabolism gets a bit "lazy." It gets the easiest out of all nutrients to use, which is why carbs are so addictive.

Your body wants carbs because they're the fastest source of energy. Yet you still eat meat and fat. When your body is only harvesting energy from carbs, the rest of the food you eat is broken down, and the energy from it is neatly stored in ever-growing fat cells since it's not being used to benefit the body. Technically, you're always hungry since the energy obtained from carbs is short-lasting, and you're getting overweight since the energy from excess calories and sugars that aren't being used is stored in your fat cells. What happens once you go on a diet?

First of all, you're bound to fail. Remember, your body is using survival mechanisms. Human biology wants you to survive, and it arguably cares less about whether or not you like the way you look. The physiological processes involved in metabolizing food are as old as mankind itself and were created in alignment with the original living conditions. Scarce food sources, lack of safe shelter, and the need to survive without eating for days at a time made the human metabolism very responsive to the presence of food in your body. Going without food for days at a time meant that a primate's metabolism had to slow down and gradually burn fat deposits so that the body survives. However, this process was made for entirely different living conditions. Primates moved around constantly, hunting and eating on the go. For that reason, their bodies formed different metabolic pathways made to extract energy from different foods and sources within the body. Why is that a problem for a modern human, and what does it have to do with dieting?

First and foremost, we're not nearly as active as our ancestors, and we live in an environment that doesn't secure clean food. Foods are saturated with sugars, additives, hormones, dyes, aromas, and pesticides. All of these substances aren't natural to the human body, and the effect of the toxic substances in food also harms your health and your metabolism. When you go on any typical diet, you aren't doing what's necessary to again spark the metabolic processes needed to burn fat. You're reducing calories, to which your body responds by slowing down your metabolism, as well as energy expenditure. If you attempt to eat less and be more active, your body's response becomes even worse. Not only does your metabolism slow down, but due to increased activity, your body begins to burn the energy from the muscle tissues, again leaving the fat stores intact. Naturally, you can suffer this malnourishment for only a little while before you dismiss the diet. Given that your metabolism is slower, once you return to your usual eating habits, the excess of blood sugar and insulin that's created from metabolizing carbs, once again, starts to fuel your fat cells. You're not replenishing the tissues that have been damaged in the process. Your metabolism remains slower, and it further slows down with each diet you attempt while the damage to your muscle tissues increases.

Given that you already tend to lose muscle tissue over the age of 50, fad diets can be detrimental. Even worse, months and years of dieting cause your hunger hormone ghrelin to increase, making you hungrier throughout the day, while leptin, the satiety hormone that's supposed to be excreted when you eat, reduces. In simple words, you are consistently hungrier over time and have more difficulty feeling full, all while your metabolism proceeds to slow down. Now, with slowing metabolism and arguably more eating as a result of the hormonal imbalance, you steadily gain weight. The unfortunate cycle of weight gain seems impossible to break unless you get your blood sugar in check and adapt your diet to a healthier, sustainable eating regimen that "reassures" your body that you'll have enough food to get by.

A part of this metabolic damage starts to resolve once you get prescribed treatment for insulin resistance or diabetes, depending on your health condition. The therapy you're taking significantly reduces harmful influences, and most people start to see improvements in the months following their life-changing doctor's appointment. Yet, without a permanent lifestyle change, any progress achieved with medication won't stick. Unless you start to fast and allow your body to gently and gradually shift metabolic processes, your health will deteriorate further despite medication.

Now, an undeniable truth is that you need to eat fewer calories than you burn to lose weight. So, what's the trick with fasting? With your usual carb-saturated diet, you technically eat more than you eat. The sheer amount of insulin released while eating is disproportionate to the food you eat and can almost be interpreted as additional calories, given that the excess of it is stored in fat cells. Yet your calorie expenditure doesn't only come from daily activities. Ha! Now we're getting to a really fun place.

You need your daily meals to fuel the ongoing mental and physical activity, which consumes energy immediately, and the hunger you feel is mostly due to that expenditure. Yet, the bulk of your daily calorie spending simply goes on survival or the support of your organs and tissues. You can, without much discomfort, reduce calorie intake only by a little and consequently "eat even less" as your body is no longer producing excess insulin that fuels your fat cells. If you're overweight, your body is burning decent amounts of calories while resting. On average, your daily calorie spending is at a minimum of 1,500 calories, which further increases with your height and weight. So only by normalizing your diet and soothing down that excess insulin production can you start to be at a calorie deficit.

Intermittent fasting further helps this process as your daily calorie spending doesn't only depend on the needs of your body but also your metabolism speed. In a fasted state, fat burning is gradually activated and intensified as hours go by, further speeding up your metabolism and creating even more calorie deficit (the difference between the number of calories you eat and those you burn.)

Your meal sizes don't need to reduce dramatically for this mechanism to take effect. You still need between 1,200 and 1,800 calories taken through food, but ideally in the form of fat, protein, and healthy fiber. Why? Because these foods keep you fuller. The same number of calories taken as carbs keeps you full, much less than a comparable number of calories from protein. It takes much more time for your body to break down protein and fats, and that keeps you full longer. The energy from your foods is now being used for intended purposes and not being directed back into the fatty supplies.

You can use this knowledge to further reflect on your perception of eating and hunger. You might think that you have to significantly reduce your food intake to lose weight, but that's not the case. This is why most dieticians recommend cutting down your daily food intake by no more than 200 calories when losing. It's barely a snack, but it's enough to lose weight dramatically over time.

FIVE PRINCIPLES OF INTERMITTENT FASTING

Intermittent fasting sounds amazing! You get to eat healthfully and in sufficient amounts. You get to enjoy the foods you like, as long as the food you're choosing is clean and healthy. You can choose between balanced, low-carb, or keto, as long as your food choices meet your nutritional needs. By now, you've learned how fasting affects your body and why your previous diets failed. After all, what you were doing with fads was growing fat while losing muscle mass. At the age of 50 and afterward, this is detrimental. You need to do the best you can to preserve your muscles, which means that you need plenty of fats and lean protein.

Yet your journey may not be as easy as you hoped it would. After all, years of metabolic damage left your body "hooked" on sugars and carbs, and quitting "cold turkey" ought to get uncomfortable. You'll go through a period of adjustment, during which your body will fight hard to get you to binge on junk food. After all, that's the easiest way to get calories and energy. Success with intermittent fasting depends on abiding by the following principles (Walters, 2021):

#1: Attainable/Realistic Schedule

You might feel like eating only once a day is the best way for you to lose weight, but is it realistic for your daily schedule? Too many times, people choose an extreme fast or attempt to fast for over 24 hours when they haven't fasted at all before. Attempting to fast too extreme or too soon might drive you away from fasting overall. When making your fasting schedule, consider the following:

- **How many hours are you active?**

An eight-hour feeding window is much easier compared to a four-hour eating window for someone who lives a busy lifestyle. Think about those times of the day when you tend to feel the hungriest and most energy-deprived, and make sure to include those times in your eating window. When it comes to longer fasts, don't attempt to fast for over 24 hours until you get used to daily fasting. A realistic fasting schedule also means adjusting fasting times to your sleep schedule. It might appear as if fasting means that you get to eat whenever you want, as long as it's during the intended feeding window. However, that's not always the case. Eating too close to your bedtime might cause you to have problems falling asleep, so make sure to be done eating at least a couple of hours before going to bed.

- **Do you have the time to rest?**

Coping with hunger can be much easier if your fasting hours are during the time of the day when you can rest and relax. Try to fit your fasting schedule so that the fasting state, which might otherwise induce hunger, matches with your free time to go out and socialize. That way, you'll have enough time to do fun activities when you get hungry, and you'll have an easier time controlling your appetite. Be careful not to get too hungry at work or when you're supposed to be highly concentrated on your activities (e.g., handwork, driving, etc.)

- **Your health/medication.**

You might need to eat before or after taking medication. Or your medicine may create the kind of side effect that requires a bit more satiating meal. Always prioritize your health and adjust the fasting schedule to your therapy. Talk to your doctor before you start fasting and let them know of your intention. If your physician thinks it's a good idea, let them recommend the ideal hours for you to be without food. If your physician recommends additional dietary restrictions, adhere to these as well. Sometimes, certain foods can interact with medications, and it becomes necessary to exclude them from your diet.

#2: *Hydration*

Drinking enough water while fasting is necessary for several reasons:

- **Helps Control Hunger.** As you found out earlier, drinking enough water helps quell hunger. If you feel like you're struggling during your fasting hours, drink a glass or two of water. Filling your stomach will help you feel less hungry, and extra hydration helps your overall health.
- **Helps Flush Out Toxins.** Fasting helps your body detox. Your tissues and organs will begin expelling all of the harmful substances from food that have piled up over the years. However, for the toxins to leave your body permanently, it's necessary to drink enough water. Hydration helps flush out toxins through your kidneys, which in return, speeds up your weight loss.
- **Helps Break Down and Remove Fat.** Similar to toxins from your blood, your body needs a way to flush out broken-down fats. You need enough water in your system so that your liver

and kidneys perform well at their jobs. This is one of the main reasons why hydration and weight loss go hand-in-hand.

- **Preserves Cardiovascular Health.** Changing your dietary habits can put extra strain on your body. If you have cardiovascular issues while trying to lose weight, it's important to drink enough water. Substances commonly found in drinking water help balance blood pressure so that you experience fewer uncomfortable changes during this transformative change.

- **Relieves Muscle and Joint Pain.** Minerals in water help relax muscles, which, in turn, can help heal and recover inflamed muscles and joints. We often think that water alone has health benefits. Oftentimes, the nutrients found in water, including minerals and electrolytes that are otherwise scarce in food, play a more essential role in body healing than those found in food. This is often the case since it's a lot easier for your body to absorb said nutrients from water than it is from food.

#3: Sleep

Sleep is universally necessary to live a healthy life, and it directly relates to weight loss. A part of why sleep is so important to lose weight is the fact that sleep deprivation contributes to weight gain. It disrupts your body's biological clock, disrupts hormonal balance, and puts your body in a state of distress. As your stress hormones spike, your body feels overall "upset." Sleep-deprived individuals have higher levels of hunger hormones throughout the day compared to people who have enough sleep.

Eating is your body's first and foremost way of coping with any kind of distress for many reasons. Throughout human evolution, food shortage has been the primary source of distress, aside from a lack of safety. The second reason behind this link is psychological. Sleep deprivation causes you to be more emotionally and mentally sensitive. You simply find it more difficult to resist food cravings. Paired with sleep deprivation, the stress of an average workday can make you feel too tired to go on. What do you do when you feel exhausted but still have to carry on with your day? You eat!

Healthy sleep, on the other hand, contributes to balancing your blood sugar and makes it easier to cope with your appetite. It gives you more physical and mental strength and energy, which further helps maximize the effects of your diet and exercise.

#4: Physical Activity

Similar to sleep, physical activity has twofold benefits to successful weight loss:

Psychological/Motivational. Sufficient physical activity, whether working out in a gym, jogging, or training in your favorite sport, stimulates relaxing and otherwise beneficial hormones like oxytocin, melatonin, and endorphins. If you haven't exercised regularly, you might feel a bit uncomfortable the first couple of times. However, over time, you'll start to feel more rested and energized. If you've been coping with depression and mood issues, exercise will help you stabilize your mood and feel better about yourself. Exercise also helps form healthy habits. It can help shift your attention away from food and toward other fun activities that support your health and weight loss.

Calorie Burning. Working out and being physically active further speeds up your metabolic rates. It helps grow your muscles and tissues, which all need extra energy. This energy is derived from fat. In this sense, exercise can further amplify the already sped-up calorie burning due to fasting and ketosis.

#5: Mindful Eating

Begin thinking more about the importance of food for your body. While it is recommended to pay attention to calories and meal compositions, a more important shift is from thinking about food as a tool to obtain comfort to a tool to obtain health. In that sense, you should:

- **Learn more about food.** Collect the dietary tips that you've gotten from your doctor and learn what makes them so beneficial for your health. Then, start learning more about what you want to achieve with your diet. Do this by learning the scientific background of healthy eating. Too often, people try to change their habits without knowing how exactly good habits work. Getting to know the principles of healthy eating per se helps you understand the effects that food has on your body. This knowledge further helps you plan meals, understand how to accurately mix, prep, store, and cook food, and craft meals that will be both delicious and healthy.

- **Get to know your taste and preferences.** Your food choices matter. A part of why you might be overeating might be the fact that you're eating more out of habit and without a thought about whether or not you enjoy the foods eaten. Take some time and go over different meal plans, recipes, and food lists. Single out the healthy foods you like the most and start tailoring your diet plan around them.

- **Write out and plan your eating schedule.** Based on the earlier reading, you should plan your eating schedule at least a week ahead. Having an idea about what your meals will look like ahead of time will give you a sense of control and instill confidence in your ability to follow through with the schedule.

- **Take enough time to eat.** Setting enough time aside to eat won't only enhance pleasure with eating, it will give you enough time to indulge in all different flavors and textures, and the meal itself will feel more satiating as a result. Furthermore, eating your meal for 20 minutes or longer helps you eat less. How? Your brain takes a while to detect that your stomach is feeling full. As this happens, your level of leptin, the satiety hormone, begins to elevate. You'll start feeling fuller while you eat, which reduces the risk of overeating. On the other hand, if you eat too fast, you might eat a lot more food than you need, simply because your brain doesn't get enough time to detect satiety.

As you can see, intermittent fasting is so much more than a diet. It is a lifestyle since it involves many different habits that train you to abstain from eating. Plus, learning how to fast also means learning how to cook and eat so that you're able to abstain from food. Lastly, intermittent fasting is a lifestyle since weight loss is only among its many benefits. Perhaps, the health and vitality that you'll regain with fasting become even more important and beneficial than the amount of weight you lost. Fasting helps prevent life-threatening illnesses and supports your body's healing. It helps you achieve lasting longevity and vitality.

6

SHOULD I WORK OUT WITHOUT EATING BREAKFAST?

Earlier in the book, we discussed if having breakfast is an "absolute must" to stay healthy. Most people are raised to believe that they need to have breakfast as early in the day as possible for a healthy life. Yet this is another legacy of past times when people ate a lot for breakfast because they'd spend long days in physical labor. Oftentimes, they wouldn't get a chance to take a break and eat before late afternoon or even evening. We don't live in those times, do we? Now we can eat on the go and take hour-long lunch breaks where we can munch on pre-made meals or take a quick trip to the nearest diner. This means we no longer need to have breakfast unless it's necessary.

DO YOU NEED BREAKFAST TO WORK OUT WITH INTERMITTENT FASTING?

The answer to this question would be "Yes" if the morning was the most labor-intensive time of your day. If your career or lifestyle is such that you're most active in the morning and then your activities gradually reduce during the day, then having a rich breakfast is a good idea. This also applies if you're working at a job where you don't have time for a lunch break, and you won't get a chance to eat again for the next five to eight hours.

If you have time for a lunch break or your lifestyle is more flexible, and you can eat at your desired time, then you can skip breakfast. What does this have to do with working out? Most people either work out before going to work or on the way back. If you're not going to work, chances are that you're adjusting your exercise routine to your other chores and errands. Naturally, working out when plenty of hours have passed since your last meal can be challenging, less in terms of health and more in terms of your mood to exercise. Although not mandatory, exercising is advisable for all age groups as it keeps your body in good shape. Exercise keeps your muscles well-developed. Microtears in muscle tissue occurs when you exercise, and as they heal, more muscle tissue grows. That way, you can slow down and prevent significant muscle loss. Furthermore, exercise keeps your joints flexible and well-lubricated. This prevents joint pain and helps promote lasting vitality.

WHY PEOPLE FEAR HUNGER

From time to time, you may find yourself in a situation of having to exercise before you have your first meal of the day. You might have your doubts about working out on an empty stomach. What if you get sick and injure yourself? Or you might even fear that strain could harm your metabolism and push your body "over the edge," causing your metabolism to slow down even further. Luckily, you don't have to worry about this with intermittent fasting. If you're keeping up a healthy eating regimen where you're getting enough calories and healthy nutrients, working out on an empty stomach shouldn't be a problem. You should only consider switching your eating window to include breakfast if you feel that working out after a busy workday would be too much. For example, if you wish your last meal in the day to be around 6-7 p.m., and your high-intensity workout session is sometime before, you should have a nourishing lunch beforehand. But, if you haven't had the time for lunch, and you expect something similar to happen in the future, then you should have your breakfast.

THE BIOLOGY OF FASTED EXERCISE

Now, let's explain a bit further why exercising in a fasted state shouldn't be a problem. You won't lose muscle mass if you exercise in a fasted state because, if you remember from your earlier reading, your muscles are getting quite a bit of nutrition when you're not eating. The slow-burning proteins, fats, and fiber from yesterday are being digested and processed in your system, sending timely energy supplies to sustain your muscles. Furthermore, if you've been fasting for a couple of weeks, your ketosis and autophagy are already underway. Your body can now "feed itself" using the already existing fat supplies. In that sense, working out in the fasted state can be even more beneficial for weight loss, as you're increasing calorie burning and burning more fat.

Studies support this, as they've established that people who fasted between 16 and 24 hours haven't lost any muscle mass due to exercise (Tamber, 2022). While you're unlikely to lose any muscle mass with exercise regardless of how you eat, studies have shown that people who eat high-protein diets have the best weight loss and exercise outcomes. If you wish to maximize the effects of exercise while fasting, and at the same time feel fuller during your fasting state, you should increase the protein in your diet. Although fasting is universally good for your body, even when exercising, some fear and doubt still remain regarding high-intensity training in the fasted state.

WHY COMBINE INTERMITTENT FASTING WITH HIIT?

A woman over 50 lifting weights on an empty stomach is a notion that most people find hard to believe. You might fear that you'll get sick and injure yourself. What if your hands start to shake, and you lose your balance and fall. It's funny how people are taught to fear that something terrible will happen to them if they don't eat. It's almost as if having an empty stomach is a potentially life-threatening situation.

What if I told you that fear of "what could happen" due to hunger is more prevalent in the obese than in healthy-weight people? This fear has several potential causes. Perhaps, you have had bad experiences in the past when you didn't eat on time. Maybe you skipped a meal and felt fatigued. If something happened as a result of that, you perhaps fell down or dropped something, this fear can start to kick in.

Remember, fasting isn't a starvation diet. You shouldn't fear negative consequences for not eating because you are already fed—or at least you should be.

If you eat as recommended in this book, you'll have plenty of strength and energy to go about your day. Exercising won't be a problem since your body is supported by rich amounts of lean meats, dairy, and veggies that you ate earlier.

This isn't the same as going hungry on a regular, imbalanced diet. Perhaps you previously ate too many carbs. The calories that you got from them didn't feed or energize your body. All of the excess energy that didn't get used momentarily got stored in your fat cells. It's not like that with a healthy diet.

A healthy diet, one that includes and emphasizes healthy protein and fat, keeps your body energized longer. Energy from meat and fat is released slowly. You might think that your stomach is empty right after you get up, but it's not. The healthy meal you had the night before is still getting digested, and that "leftover" energy will support your body as you work out.

Yet, if you look at intermittent fasting communities, you'll find a lot of empowering examples of women who, indeed, do high-intensity workouts while having fasted for over 14 or 16 hours. Granted, the idea might sound a bit extreme, especially if you haven't been exercising much as of late or you haven't exercised at all. No matter how much is said in the media about the importance of exercise and how many times physicians recommend exercising to their patients, workouts seem to be the weakest link on the list of priorities. First comes work and family, then chores and errands, while social life and hobbies remain a privilege that most people are unwilling to sacrifice at the expense of working out. Yet, as years pass and medical bills start to pile up, most people of mature age start to regret not taking enough time to exercise. Don't be this person! You can start turning your life around regardless of age, and yes, you can enjoy high-intensity training even if you're over 50 and while fasting.

As demonstrated in research, intermittent fasting makes for a great combo with high-intensity interval training (HIIT) for all age groups. Now, just the phrase "high-intensity" alone can be intimidating. You may start thinking like you're expected to binge like a weight-lifting state champion, but that's not the case. Not to say you wouldn't make it if you wanted to, but that's a topic for another book.

High-intensity interval training consists of short, intense workouts combined with breaks. The benefits of HIIT for women over 50 include

- improved general health
- better mood and sleep regulation
- ease of pre-menopause and menopause symptoms
- better shape and flexibility
- reduced risks of metabolic and cardiovascular illnesses (Batitucci et al., 2022)

A good instructor can help you discover amazing HIIT workouts that will help you burn through belly fat within months and give you a more youthful appearance. If you still lack faith in HIIT, just run a quick Google search and see the transformations of women over 50 with HIIT. Wow! Just at first glance, you can notice that the women's faces look tighter, which can be attributed to the hormonal and detoxifying benefits of these exercises. If you thought that weight fluctuations have left your skin stretched out permanently and you'll have to cope with it, it turns out you're wrong. Skin can indeed tighten with HIIT and to an amazing degree.

If you're starting to feel motivated to try out HIIT, wait until you hear what it does to your body when combined with fasting. Studies found that doing high-intensity interval workouts in a fasted state can improve your overall health, body composition, and quality of life. This is essential if you're recovering from obesity, as well as if you're in the range of healthy weight and you simply wish to tighten up.

Women who participated in studies and exercised in combination with intermittent fasting saw the following improvements:

- increased metabolic rate (faster metabolism and fat burning)
- a four percent loss in body fat with a two percent increase in muscle mass
- improved strength and aerobic capacity (Batitucci et al., 2022)

Overall, doing high-intensity workouts while fasting helped women improve strength and aerobic capacity, which had been demonstrated by visible weight loss. However, for your exercises to be successful, you must work with a professional instructor. High-intensity exercises draw a lot of energy and can be too much if you're doing them on your own and without proper guidance. However, if you're fasting and you want to increase health benefits, don't let training intimidate you. Professional instructors will take all relevant factors into account, including your age, shape, body composition, schedule, lifestyle, and health, before designing an exercise program. If you're inexperienced with high-intensity exercise, your instructor will start you on light exercises and then increase their intensity gradually. If you opt in for professional training, you shouldn't fear discomfort or injury. You can simply push your body further and slowly build up strength as you rejuvenate your look and replenish your health.

BENEFITS OF WORKING OUT WHILE FASTED

If done properly, exercising in a fasted state, particularly in ketosis, helps you build muscles, replenish your health, and rejuvenate your look. This may come as a shock to anyone thinking that you should never exercise without having a meal beforehand. That is not to say that this assumption isn't rooted in truth, though. People who eat regular balanced or high protein diets may indeed lose some muscle mass if working out on an empty stomach. However, this doesn't apply to fasting, given that you otherwise eat a healthful diet that's rich or high in protein.

Opposed to fearing that fasting exercises might harm your muscles is the belief that fasting, particularly supported by ketosis and autophagy, makes exercise more effective. The goals of exercise are many. Exercise stretches, flexes, and relaxes your body, which improves your blood circulation and cardiovascular health and reduces joint pain. Since your joints are a curious medley of bone, muscle, tendons, and blood vessels, a lack of physical activity can greatly harm them. The less you move, the less blood circulates through your joints. When you exercise, you move your joints so that they're getting their healthy blood supply. This helps keep other tissues in your joints healthy as well. Reduced circulation through your joints also means that they aren't getting enough nutrition, so the process of aging is faster. Another important benefit of exercise is that it helps grow and maintain your muscle mass, as exercising in a fasted state leverages peaks of growth hormone and enhances your endurance capacity.

Still, if you'd look at what researchers have to say on this topic, you'd find diverse opinions that all emphasize certain benefits and shortcomings when it comes to choosing whether to exercise in a fasted or fed state. Before we start reflecting on whether you should be hungry or full when exercising, let's briefly address the diversity of priorities, goals, and exercise effects that researchers have in mind when doing their studies. Exercise serves more than one purpose. For some, the main purpose is weight loss and weight maintenance. Other women, not all, also find it important to boost endurance and flexibility. While some women care deeply about growing muscle mass, others are more interested in the mental and even spiritual aspects of movement and exercise. There's no uniform opinion when it comes to exercising and intermittent fasting simply because people have different priorities with exercise. Knowing this, you can start to reflect on the benefits of fasting for exercise in the following aspects:

Fat Burning and Ketosis

As demonstrated by previous research, exercising while fasting helps you burn fat more effectively. If you combine fasting with the keto diet, fat burning only increases. Studies demonstrate that you can expect between two and four percent more fat loss if you pair exercise with fasting, especially with obesity. If you're obese and decide to include workouts in your weekly regimen, adjustments are needed to keep your regimen safe and prevent harm while exercising. Some risks for obese women who start to exercise include injury and hypoglycemia. The first can occur due to sudden muscle and joint strain, while the latter happens as you're still looking for that sweet spot between eating enough to be energized and maintaining a calorie deficit. Fasting helps in this regard as it supports healing processes. It also balances blood sugar, reducing the risks of suddenly feeling sick while exercising.

Strength and Endurance

Working out while fasting can feel like you're adding strain to your body, but that's not the case. On the outside, you might be "starving" since you haven't had a meal before exercise. But on the inside, your body is slowly being fed energy from the day before. This energy provides strength for you to exercise. Your muscles and tissues, on the other hand, receive fuel from the fat burning. If you recall from the first chapters of this book, another benefit of fasting is that you shift to a fat-burning metabolic pathway, which starts to release energy from your fat cells and direct it into muscles. In that sense, you're doing just the right thing to promote fat burning: you're providing a demand for your muscles to draw energy from your fat cells, which causes your body to literally "suck out" fat to grow and heal itself.

Endurance, on the other hand, is a measure of how much strain your cardiovascular system can endure. The better endurance you have, the better your cardiovascular health. Aside from having more strength and energy for your daily activities, endurance promotes lasting longevity as it keeps your blood vessels strong and healthy.

Improved Hormonal Balance

Exercise while fasting means doubling the dosage of human growth hormone (HGH) released into your body. You might think this hormone promotes tissue growth, but this isn't the case. Tissues grow by multiplying healthy cells, and they spend energy from fat. HGH promotes converting fatty acids and glucose into energy, which then goes into muscles, the heart, lungs, and other organs.

DOWNSIDES AND RISKS OF EXERCISE IN A FASTED STATE

Neither exercise nor fasting is a "one-size-fits-all" regimen. Both will ideally become your lifestyle, but adjustments are needed to find routines that benefit your body and mind. Too intense fasting paired with overly straining exercise can have harmful effects, including:

Performance

If your body isn't fed in the wholesome sense of the word while you exercise, your workouts may not be as effective. With intermittent fasting, the number of calories and your meal composition affect your tomorrow, not your today. In this sense, you should eat more calories and protein the day before than the morning before your workout.

Mood and Stress

Exhaustion from too much exercise on an empty stomach can make you feel grumpy and stressed out. On a busy day, mental and physical strain can deplete your motivation to exercise. Releasing stress hormones while working out isn't good for your health either. If you have mood disorders paired with health conditions like obesity, exhausting yourself too much can do more harm than good.

Health Risks

Adjustments to your diet and exercise are due to your weight, health, and history of injury (if any). Overly intense exercise can put you at risk for hypoglycemia and cardiac problems, so ensure that your instructor has a thorough knowledge of which workout adjustments you need.

Luckily, there are numerous ways to adjust your diet and exercise routine if you plan on combining intermittent fasting and exercise (which you should). These adjustments include

Caloric Intake

Calculate your ideal caloric intake if you're fasting and exercising. Do this simply by calculating your daily caloric expenditure while accounting for your height, weight, and age and deducing the number of calories needed for an optimal calorie deficit. Next, consult your training instructor regarding the exercises you should do to achieve the desired weight effects and apply the dietary adjustment to your recommended daily calories. That way, you get a clear picture of how much you should eat while fasting to maintain a calorie deficit and to be fed enough to exercise.

Exercise Adjustment

Your choice of exercise depends on the results you wish to achieve. Typical workout goals include weight loss, muscle tightening or growth in certain areas, or more endurance, flexibility, and others. Yet, some of these goals are more important to you than others. With obesity, women prioritize fat burning and muscle preservation, paired with tightening, to achieve their desired shape. Fitness instructors often share the same opinion and only recommend starting to do more intense exercises for muscle growth and endurance after you've met the desired health and weight goals. However, your exercises should be personalized and well-adjusted to your health and weight goals. Your instructor should adjust exercises in regard to:

- **your current health and weight.** You might need a variety of common exercises to support cardiovascular performance and prevent muscle and joint injury.
- **your health.** Certain medical conditions affect which exercises you should and shouldn't do. Your instructor should be knowledgeable about

whether or not you should include cardio exercises and weightlifting, as these workouts are known to cause too much strain with some medical conditions (e.g., sciatica, herniated disk, arrhythmia, and others).

- **your goals.** Break down your exercise and weight goals with your instructor. Give them a simple description of how you want your body to look once the exercises start to take effect. For example, you can tell them that you want a more prominent behind and a thinner waist. Maybe having your abs visible isn't as important to you as it is to tighten your arms. The more your instructor knows about the look that you wish to achieve with exercises, the better they're able to help you.

Fasting Adjustment

Fasting gives you all the choices regarding whether you wish to work out in the fasted state, during your feeding hours, or right before or after a meal. None of these will harm your body. But your choice of time to work out will affect the results if paired with fasting. You'll arguably see more fat burning and weight loss if exercising in the fasted state. But, if you wish to start "buffing up" and further growing your muscles and endurance, you can shift to working out closer to eating. Sometimes, pairing fast and fitness is less a matter of choice and more dependent on possibilities. Your work and schedule might dictate when you'll fast and when to eat, and in this case, you should place your workouts at a fasting time that best promises to achieve the desired goal.

As you can see, there's not much risk associated with exercising while fasting. Unless your physicians advise against it, there's no reason why you shouldn't give high-intensity workouts a shot. Working out while fasting won't put your body under extreme strain, nor will it, under normal circumstances, make you feel sick.

7

ORGANIZE YOUR DAY

By now, you've learned how to start fasting, what to expect, and how to cope with different challenges that might present themselves. Success with intermittent fasting, to a great degree, depends on how well you organize your day.

CHOOSE YOUR IDEAL FASTING REGIMEN

If you're just starting with fasting, your first steps to making a successful schedule include several different eating patterns, from easiest to hardest:

16/8 Fasting and Its Variations

This fasting pattern is the most common. It includes an eight-hour window followed by fasting for the next sixteen hours. For example, if you had breakfast at 8 a.m., your dinner should be no later than 4 p.m. Then, you shouldn't eat anything until 8 a.m. the next morning. This is often the easiest fasting regimen to follow. However, if you choose this lifestyle, think about your ideal eating time. Although finishing your dinner early and pausing until the next breakfast is thought to yield the fastest fat loss, you'll be successful on any other timeline as long as you take a 16-hour break between meals. If you find it too difficult to go this long without food, you can choose a 14/10 fast, which leaves you with a 10-hour eating window. However, if you wish to intensify your fast, you can reduce your eating window to six hours and extend your fast to eighteen hours. As you get used to this way of eating, you can narrow down your eating window to four hours and extend the fast to twenty hours.

Some studies done on mice showed that this method of fasting helped make their bodies more resilient to diabetes, inflammation, liver disease, and obesity. However, there are different views regarding whether you should focus on the total number of calories or a specific diet. Still, even without major dietary adjustments, studies hint that you should be able to lose weight. Here are some tips for successful 16:8 fasting:

- **Delay breakfast as much as possible.** Most women have intense cravings in the evening. If your last meal for the day is set before 5 p.m., it's possible that the later cravings will be too hard to handle. If you have your breakfast at noon, your dinner will fall sometime around 8 p.m. This schedule still keeps you within the recommended feeding window, and it's less likely that you'll break your fast with a snack.

- **Keep water close.** The advice to hydrate as much as possible is found frequently in this book. It serves to remind you of the role that hydration has on your weight loss and overall health. Keep a bottle of water close to you at all times, as water prolongs the sensation of satiety. Have one glass of water before your meal, one after, and at least one or two between meals. Aside from helping you feel full, water also helps flush out and metabolize carbs and fats.

- **Have your carbs in the morning.** The experiences of women at the beginning of their intermittent fasting journey show that each time of the day is challenging for different reasons. You need more energy in the morning, a pick-me-up in the afternoon, and then a satisfying meal toward the evening to cope with late-night cravings. However, many women go about this the wrong way. If you have a fuller breakfast, you'll reach the end of the day with fewer calories left within your daily limit. Instead, start with a light breakfast, and allow for more of your allocated carbs. Then, have more meaty and fatty meals later in the day to keep you full until the next morning.

If you "clean up" your diet of unhealthy, processed foods and you keep your macronutrient ratio within the recommended scope, you should start losing weight within the first couple of weeks. After you've gotten used to this form of fasting, you can progress to more intense fasting methods.

5/2 Weekly Fasting

This fasting pattern entails that you fast at your selected pace for five days of the week and then have two low-calorie days throughout the week. Every two or three days, you should limit your food intake to no more than 500 calories. You should consult your physician before reducing your calories to below 1000 to avoid negative health consequences. If you feel like you'd benefit from a day or two of weekly calorie restriction, follow these useful guidelines:

- **Space out your fasting days.** Always have at least one non-restricted day between the two days of fasting with calorie restriction. This gives your body enough time to recover, feed, and replenish. Severe calorie restriction for two days in a row might be too much.

- **Shuffle your fasting days.** Avoid fasting on the same days of the week. Your body benefits from being "tricked" with fasting and having to use all of its beneficial healing processes to compensate for the lack of calories. If you fast on the same days of the week, your metabolic system will begin to adapt. Plus, you want to avoid marking some days of the week as "calorie restriction days." This could reflect poorly on your quality of life and fasting satisfaction.

- **Prepare for fasting.** You should ideally take a look at your schedule and choose the least stressful days to fast. For example, if you expect to have a busy week, then you can fast on Monday and Saturday. Most people feel more energized on Mondays than on other days of the week, and if you don't work weekends, there will be less physical and mental strain on your fasting day. Similarly, if your schedule suddenly opens up, and you feel like you'll be able to afford a slower day, you can choose to fast.

- **Consider exercising.** There are both benefits and risks associated with exercise on your fasting days. You might benefit from faster fat burning but also be at risk for greater muscle loss. The choice of whether or not to exercise on your calorie restriction days is entirely on you. If you feel like you'll benefit from working out while fasting, and you don't mind a bit more hunger than usual, then go for it! Remember, when you exercise in a fasted state, you burn fat faster, and your cardiovascular system becomes more resilient. However, if there's a medical need for you to slow down and avoid exercise during your fasting days, feel free to do so.

A Single-Meal Diet

Often called the "Warrior diet," this pattern means that you only get to eat once a day. However, eating once a day doesn't necessarily mean that you need to go hungry. You can plan your single meal carefully and make sure that it contains the exact number of calories and nutrient composition that you're looking for. Furthermore, it's recommended to extend your meal to a full hour, during which you'll eat slowly and mindfully. While this does seem like the most extreme version of intermittent fasting, it gets a lot easier after a couple of days. You can eat a single meal in a day by having one larger dinner after another. However, both meals still need to satisfy your nutritive needs for the day.

Eating only one meal a day can sound intimidating, but it's not that difficult. If you plan your diet for the day carefully, you shouldn't experience a lot of discomfort. Here's what you can do to be more successful with this method of fasting:

- **Emphasize fats and protein.** If you choose this diet, you'll go almost 24 hours without blood sugar to keep you going. Don't ruin this by eating too many carbs! While you should include healthy carbs in your chosen/recommended amount, keep your meal fatty and meaty. Meals that are saturated with carbs won't keep you full for the entire next day. Instead, they'll get metabolized into sugar quickly, leaving you with that awkward morning hunger and an entire day to go by without food.
- **Be mindful of calories!** While some experts on intermittent fasting say that you can have as many calories as you want with this diet and

still lose weight, most are against it. The overwhelming majority of experts agree that you might hurt your weight loss by eating everything uncontrollably. The best-recommended meal is the one consisting of the number of calories, meats, veggies, and fats, in your usual recommended ratio.

- **Drink coffee and water.** Keep feeling fuller during the day by drinking plenty of liquids. Coffee, in particular, will quell your appetite for a few more hours and help you fast until your next meal.

- **Make time fly by.** The best way to go an entire day without eating is to make a schedule that doesn't leave time or possibility to eat. This can be tricky depending on your job, but it's not impossible. For example, you can schedule these intense fasting days if you're planning to spend a day outside. Do you know how you sometimes feel too tired to eat? Spending the day in the fresh air can make it easier to abstain from food until dinner.

- **Remove temptations.** Think about the potential negative influences that could drive you to break your fast and eat when you shouldn't be eating. Do your coworkers bring treats to work? Then decide to spend the day in the office or work from home. If you live with other people who aren't fasting, have their food packaged separately in the fridge to remind you not to touch it. If possible, remove all food just for the day. You can clear out your fridge and either freeze or give away everything that you won't be eating until dinner.

Alternate Day Fasting

This fasting regimen is quite similar to eating a single meal a day. Except, it's not a constant way of eating, but instead a periodic fast that you use every other day. For example, you can eat a regular diet on Monday and then not eat anything until the night of the following Tuesday. The next day, you can continue using your selected eating regimen. This way of eating can be easier than the single-meal diet if you're finding it difficult to eat only once a day for a long time. However, it can also be difficult since you're making a switch between eating however you want and not eating anything at all.

If you don't wish to abstain from food completely with alternate day fasting, you can opt for a 500-calorie diet or a liquid diet during this time. While studies support the premise that you can lose weight effectively with this form of fasting, it might not be for people whose medical condition doesn't support going without food for the entire day or having very little calories. This could be the case with cardiovascular diseases and diabetes, as well as any other illness that could contribute to getting sick while fasting.

If your physician supports and allows alternate day fasting, you can give it a try! The effects of this method are supported by studies that have reported overweight adults losing over 11 pounds in three months. If you decide to try out this method, you should follow these tips for better success:

- **Calculate the exact calorie intake.** It may not be necessary to give up food completely or limit yourself strictly to the 500 recommended calories. Some experts on the topic suggest that you should limit your calorie intake to 25% of your usual calorie intake. If your recommended calories exceed 2,000, you can consider slightly boosting your meals.
- **Have an early lunch and a late dinner.** How does one go an entire (work)day with very little food? To go through the day successfully, you'll have to trick your body into feeling full. You'll do this by eating your breakfast very early. An early breakfast will elevate your blood sugar and give you the energy for the majority of the

workday. You can add a light lunch mid-day to keep you going. Your dinner should be as late as you can endure. The insulin spike that happens after eating will keep you feeling fuller throughout the evening, which will make it easier to cope until the next morning.

- **Have early meals and fast for the rest of the day.** If you're not struggling with late-night appetite, you should ideally have early meals and extend your fast until the next morning.

BREAKING YOUR FAST? HERE'S HOW TO GO ABOUT IT

Great job on deciding to fast and for considering going without food for 24 hours or longer! If you follow all of the instructions given in this book, you should be able to do so without much discomfort or risk to your health. As important as it is to find the right way to fast, it's equally important how you're breaking your fast if you spent a full day or longer without food.

Finding the best method for breaking your fast maximizes the benefits of going so long without food and reduces the discomfort that might happen if your first meal after fasting is too heavy on the stomach.

It's important to remember that, even if you break your fast before you planned, you shouldn't beat yourself up over it. The ability to fast for longer times, to a large degree, depends on what you ate before fasting. If your pre-fast meal wasn't satiating enough, and particularly if it didn't contain enough fat and protein, it's possible that you simply didn't eat enough calories. If you've broken your fast sooner than you were supposed to because you started to feel dizzy or sick, it was the right decision. After all, fasting shouldn't feel agonizing and torturous. It should feel pleasant, and any food cravings you feel on your day of fasting should be explained by sugar or carb addiction, and even mode, more so than biological hunger. Any other discomfort should prompt you to take precautions and get the nutrition that you need. You should, however, take a closer look at what your previous meal looked like and consider adding a little bit more food the next time so that you're able to resist cravings again. However, this shouldn't be just any food. Prioritize lean meat and protein because it will keep you feeling full longer.

Once you've successfully fasted for a day or longer, take a careful approach to breaking your fast. Your digestive system has emptied since the last time you ate, and numerous beneficial processes were triggered in your body. The main purpose of the effort to break your fast correctly is to avoid digestive discomfort more so than prevent any health risks. Health risks associated with correct fasting are few (the emphasis being on 'correct'), and the same goes for breaking them.

Yet, using undesirable food to break your fast can affect your mood. Your hormonal system is highly responsive to food. You might feel an urge to binge on a bucket of chicken legs, but your brain won't like it. You might see a surge of nervousness and sluggishness as a result of all the hormones associated with a bad mood going into 'hyper mode.' to avoid this, follow a few simple guidelines:

Hydrate With Vinegar

A tablespoon or two of apple cider vinegar diluted in a glass of water will further promote fat burning and make you feel fuller after your meal. That way, you will eat a bit less than you normally would after a long fast, and you'll create an even bigger caloric deficit throughout the day.

Apple cider vinegar will also help you stabilize your mood thanks to its effect on hormones, and combined with a lower caloric intake, it will help you feel more energized throughout the day.

Start Your Meal on a Liquid Note

Have some bone broth. Bone broth is light, and it has a lot of minerals and nutrients that will gently spark your digestive system without burdening it. What you're trying to achieve is for the enzymes in your stomach to start working slowly, which prevents heartburn, gas, and other types of intestinal discomfort.

Bone broth also contains collagen, which benefits your skin, nails, and hair. Your body is made more sensitive and will easily absorb nutrients from liquid foods at this particular period, making it an ideal time to reap the gentle benefits of cooked foods.

Support Your Microbiome

Cleansing your digestive system of food has removed, or at least significantly reduced, many toxic substances that harmed your intestinal flora. Now, it's time to treat your intestines with nutrient-packed, fiber-rich foods that will nourish the friendly microorganisms in your stomach. Once recuperated, these organisms will contribute to producing hormones that promote a relaxed, pleasant mood, and they'll also promote immune health and weight loss.

One of my favorite first meals to have is the classic steak and eggs with a side of fruit. These foods are rich in protein, micronutrients, and fiber which will all get quickly broken down and absorbed. While the foods mentioned above feed your microbiome, some foods help seed diverse, healthy organisms.The easiest of these foods to find are fermented food. Dairy, like yogurt and soft cheeses, as well as sauerkraut, all contain safe and healthy microorganisms. Once you have these foods, believe it or not, these microorganisms take only a couple of hours to find a home in your digestive system. From there, these organisms will help synthesize beneficial nutrients and hormones and will hence benefit your health, mood, and weight loss.

The whole purpose of this fast-breaking routine is to eat light foods that won't feel too heavy on the stomach. Don't let yourself overeat due to feeling overly hungry! Simply follow general recommendations for healthy eating and savor your meal for at least 20 minutes. Ideally, stretch out your first meal to a whole hour. That way, you'll give your body enough time to start producing the satiety hormone, and you won't overeat.

TIPS TO TURN FASTING INTO A LIFESTYLE

If you're fasting between 12 and 24 hours, you'll need smart adjustments to maintain it in the long run. Let's face it, long fasting is much easier the first couple of times since it's a new experience. You might find yourself amazed by the changes you feel, and you initially have more motivation and persistence to carry out the regimen. But what happens when you wish to fast every other day or every third day? You might start to feel demotivated, and if you haven't made proper lifestyle and diet adjustments, fasting can start to feel difficult. Luckily, there are things you can do to turn your fasting regimen into a lifestyle that will become effortless over time.

A big part of creating your fasting lifestyle is in understanding how various changes are triggered in your body and how to willfully affect the exact changes that you wish to induce. Implementing the changes that give you the results you're looking for ensures satisfaction, which further boosts your motivation to carry out the lifestyle.

Here are the major principles of a fasting lifestyle:

Choose Fasting Principles to Target Health and Weight Goals

Not everyone has the same issues. Perhaps, your sleep is just fine, and you can afford to eat whenever you want in a day. Or, if you wish to burn fat more than grow muscle, you can go for longer eating windows instead of trying to confine all of your meals to a couple of hours. Go back to reading about the fasting principles in Chapter 5 and decide which of these is more important than the others. Implement lifestyle changes that affect whatever is bothering you rather than trying to inflict all changes at once.

Find Your Ideal Eating Styles

There's a variety of fasting styles to choose from. Listen to your body's cues, and feel free to try out different variations of fasting. Eating styles also need to accommodate your taste and schedule so that your meal plan becomes attainable.

Eat Prebiotics and Probiotics

Don't forget to feed your microbiome! In the previous section, you learned about how greens, cruciferous vegetables, and fermented foods can benefit your health. You can have these foods each day, and they'll both seed and feed the beneficial microorganisms in your body.

Address Your Toxins

Are you smoking, drinking too much coffee, or living in a moldy home? Fasting isn't only a matter of food. The effects of your lifestyle changes will be much better if you make sure to remove any toxins from your environment. Inspect your home and the chemicals that you use each day and see if there are any substances present in your environment that are a potential health hazard.

Consider Supplementation

It's a good idea to support more intense fasting with supplementation. Although, in theory, fasting shouldn't negatively impact your health, you can't guarantee that your diet has sufficient nutrients. However, you shouldn't take supplements long-term. Instead, take the supplement as long as you need it, and then stop when you, again, become able to get your daily nutrients from their natural sources.

Use Other Improvements

Various therapies enhance the benefits of fasting, like visiting a chiropractor, doing cryotherapy, or visiting a hyperbaric chamber or sauna. These complementing treatments further stimulate your body's healing processes and boost your health significantly.

8

CREATING A BALANCED DIET
FOR YOUR BEST RESULTS

G reat job for sticking all the way until the end and learning the ins and outs of intermittent fasting. In the previous chapter, you learned about the numerous eating patterns that you can apply. Now, you can start making decisions regarding when to eat and when to fast. Admittedly, studies demonstrate that you'll reap benefits from fasting whether or not you make dietary adjustments. However, adopting a simple, delicious, and, more importantly, attainable diet will help make a lifelong transformation. Whereas the previous chapter focused on WHEN to eat, the last chapter of your intermittent fasting manual will show you WHAT to eat. My suggestion is to consult a Registered Dietician in order to get an approved meal plan best for you. We as humans are so unique that there is no such thing as a one size fits all diet. Therefore, speaking to a professional such as a dietician will be the best option for optimal results.

WHY IS EATING HEALTHY LONG-TERM SO HARD?

Let's face it, staying healthy in middle age will require finding an easy way to eat. Your diet regimen must work whether you're sick, healthy, busy, or vacationing. You need a healthy framework for what foods to pick at celebrations and what to get in a grocery store when you have only 15 minutes to fill your fridge for the upcoming week. You won't be able to do that if you try to maintain a diet that requires you to go to five different stores or order bread online. The Mediterranean diet is a great option, and the reason for that is its ease of maintenance and accessibility, as well as proven health benefits.

Now, let's briefly reflect on why it's so hard to eat healthfully and address the real reasons why people in middle age start gaining weight suddenly:

Lack of Time

No time for healthy shopping, cooking, and eating is the biggest reason why so many women start gaining weight in middle age. At first glance, it may seem as if middle age will bring you more free time. You expect to have gained more stability in your career and more financial stability, and those with families expectedly count on their children to become more independent. Well, it turns out that middle age, if not too busy, can prove that you can have "too much of a good thing." Plenty of women are still quite engaged at work, and many also support their families. You may not be running around the same way you did in previous decades, but you now occupy yourself with other priorities. It may just turn out that the amount of time you can allocate for healthy eating is no greater than before. Eating in a rush, skipping meals, and grabbing foods from shelves frantically on the go can easily lead to overeating and consequential insulin resistance problems.

Limited Food Choices

My wild guess is that you shop for groceries in one of several stores near your home or job. Shopping from limited sources also narrows down your choices of food. If there are no available healthy foods, you have no choice but to compromise and get what's available, hoping you'll be able to get healthier options the next time. As time goes by, you're thinking less about healthy eating and more about getting the same grocery list that "works" over and over again. This is an easy trap to fall in. The fewer meal choices, the greater chances that you'll eventually turn to fried foods, pasta, and take-out.

Lack of Eating Intuition

All of the previous, when combined, negatively affect your natural appetite. You feel less biological hunger and more of the addictive yearning created by a sugar addiction and the vicious cycle of insulin resistance. While you used to crave veggies and lean meats, you now can't stop thinking about pizza wherever you get hungry. Studies demonstrate that people with a healthy eating intuition can regulate food intake quite well. They can intuitively decide on meal sizes and feel significantly less yearning for unhealthy foods. But what happened to your eating intuition? The answer is simple: sugar addiction. Eating foods saturated with chemicals and artificial flavors, which includes processed sugars, knocks your understanding of taste out of balance. You no longer sense or appreciate the fullness of healthy foods and herb spices. Instead, your mind is set on satisfying your sugar addiction. If you were to return to a healthy diet and nurture your eating intuition, you would be able to pick those foods and meal sizes that match your body's needs, which is also supported by science. You wouldn't have to rely on a chart or a program to tell you what to eat. For example, you'd feel a craving for yummy, boiled chicken breast with a little bit of cottage cheese and broccoli. You could summon the taste of foods and visualize the meal, despite not eating it. You could tell exactly how much of each food you want, and you'd find that eating it feels as satiating as you imagined.

Stress Eating

Stress sometimes manifests as appetite. In part due to biological responses to cortisol, and in part due to using food as a coping mechanism, quick sugary meals become a treat for comfort. Stress eating only makes your stress responses worse, though. In the long term, you become more prone to strong emotional reactions to issues you used to resolve easily. The more you stress-eat, the more stressed you become. As eating remains your main coping mechanism, you're failing to make the needed changes and, instead, turn to eating even more.

As you can see, you need a healthy eating solution that will work well with all situations that life can throw at you.

WHAT'S THE MEDITERRANEAN DIET AND WHY IS IT SO GREAT FOR FASTING?

As the name suggests, this diet is modeled after Mediterranean cuisine. It uses the foods that are typical for this area and combines strong flavors with interesting spices for delicious meals. When it comes to food choices, the Mediterranean diet is considered to be one of the healthiest options out there. It consists mainly of plants, with plenty of whole vegetables, fruits, grains, beans, nuts, and legumes. Your meat portions, however, are a bit less, with the diet including mainly lean protein with an emphasis on fish and seafood. You can indulge in poultry, pork, and beef, as with any other diet, but in smaller portions. Here are some of the main reasons why this diet works so well with intermittent fasting:

- **Keto-Friendly.** This diet uses a lot of fats from butter, olive oil, nuts, and fish. These foods are rich in omega-3 fatty acids and will help you nourish your body, support immune and cardiovascular health, and burn fat while staying in ketosis. Even better, using the principles of the keto diet in combination with the Mediterranean diet will yield delicious, nourishing meals, which consist of easily accessible foods that you can get in any store. As you're about to see, none of the foods used in the Mediterranean diet are considered exotic. They're quite plain, only used in ways that allow each veggie to shine.

- **High in protein.** The Mediterranean diet recommends having a piece of meat each day, with fish being included at least twice a week. You can have as much fermented dairy as you like. However, this diet limits your red meat intake to several monthly portions. Still, you can eat enough meat, dairy, and eggs to stay low-carb or keto and normalize insulin as a result. This makes the Mediterranean diet even more simple, as all of these foods are found in most grocery stores.

- **Clean and whole.** The Mediterranean diet has one thing in common with keto and intermittent fasting, and it is the love for clean eating. It recommends getting whole foods whenever possible, and the no-chemical principle is also reflected in beverage recommendations. You're advised against drinking juices, with only a couple of glasses of wine recommended weekly. However, the wine you drink should be high-quality and organic as well. You're advised to drink mostly water and plenty of it.

Choosing the Mediterranean diet as a long-term inter-mittent fasting solution is a great idea. Aside from starchy vegetables and grains that are high in carbs, you can pretty much include the foods you like as long as they're clean. This diet also eliminates processed sugars, both in meals and drinks. However, it does include fruit and honey. If you wish for a little bit of natural sugar in your diet, in the long run, you can enjoy some fruit and honey which can be extreme-ly beneficial with micronutrients and antioxidant prop-erties. You won't have to worry about eating a recommended serving of nature's candy, without fear of disrupting your insulin balance.

THE HEALTH BENEFITS OF THE MEDITERRANEAN DIET FOR MIDDLE-AGED WOMEN

Cardiovascular Health

Healthy fats, high protein and fiber, and an abundance of micronutrients that are included in this diet help women in middle age maintain cardiovascular health. This diet reduces the risk of cardiovascular disease by a whopping 25%! Some of the obvious reasons for this include:

- **Less processed sugar.** The Mediterranean diet balances your blood sugar since it excludes sugary foods. You can use healthy fruits and veggies as snacks. Most women on the Mediterranean diet opt for vegetable and fruit sticks dipped in cottage cheese with spices. With endless options for your cheese dip, there's simply no excuse to get a fast-food snack or to purchase sweets. This diet further includes amazing substitutes for flour, like beans and whole grains. Even if you decide to include carbs in your weight maintenance stage, there's less chance of gaining weight.

- **Full and satiating.** This diet includes foods that keep you full longer. Since the diet uses healthy fats, there's no need to worry about weight gain. However, you can still have your juicy slice of meat, which helps design meals for longer fasting. You'll easily combine meats and vegetables to create light-tasting meals. Yet, these meals will be both calorie-dense and weight-loss-friendly. The fats used in this diet will go straight into building your muscles and tissues, whereas those from junk food stick to your arteries and blood vessels, further endangering your health.

- **Speedy weight loss.** If your cardiovascular health is at risk due to obesity, this diet helps you lose weight promptly. Healthy weight loss significantly reduces your risks of cardiovascular disease, while weight reduction supports recovery.

The risk of cardiovascular disease significantly increases in middle age. The loss of muscle tissue, less physical activity, and slower metabolism all create unhealthy influences on your cardiovascular system. The Mediterranean diet helps address and reduce, if not eliminate, all of those negative influences.

Mental Health Benefits

Depression is a notable mental health problem for women of all ages, and it remains so in middle age. Among the many risk factors for depression, diet plays an important role. Your diet affects hormonal balance, which in turn affects your mental health.

The research discovered a definite neurological connection between your brain and your stomach called the gut-brain axis. Your food choices, if healthy, can promote the production of serotonin, endorphins, melatonin, and oxytocin. These hormones help balance your mood and better regulate your sleep. However, the synthesis of these hormones begins in your gut. If you have a healthy microbiome, your stomach does its part successfully, and you start to feel relaxed and emotionally pleased after eating a healthy meal. However, years of unhealthy eating can cause leaky gut syndrome. This syndrome occurs when chemicals from unhealthy food destroy healthy microorganisms in your gut. When this happens, you produce fewer hormones that allow you to feel relaxed and happy and begin producing more stress hormones. Why? When your gut microbiome is depleted, your gut starts passing pathogens and chemicals into the blood. This causes your immune system to become overactive. In some cases, the immune system is active constantly, which causes the production of cortisol. Similar autoimmune responses occur when your body can no longer distinguish dangerous substances from nutrients that are commonly found in the blood.

Luckily, fasting paired with the Mediterranean diet can help turn this process around. What you need to do is help the recovery of your microbiome. If you recall from earlier sections, vegetables and fermented foods both seed and feed healthy gut microorganisms. The longer you're on the Mediterranean diet, the more your microbiome recovers. You start producing more of the hormones that affect positive mood, and less of the stress hormones.

If you're coping with mood disorders and depression, rest assured that the Mediterranean diet can help. Multiple studies found improvements in patients who had clinical depression (Yin et al., 2021). Long-term, this diet can help stabilize mood regardless of age!

Better Overall Health

Women between the ages of 50 and 69 years showed signs of healthier aging when they followed a Mediterranean diet. These women increase their chances of healthy aging by over 40%! They had less risk of developing a whole range of diseases, from Parkinson's disease, osteoporosis, metabolic syndrome, and cancer to kidney disease and type 2 diabetes (Babio et al., 2009; Savanelli et al., 2017). You'll benefit your general health the most if you limit your alcohol intake and reduce red meats to the greatest possible degree.

This is great news for women who enjoy fish and seafood. You can eat more fish paired with veggies and grains and season your delicious meals with numerous herbs and spices. These tasty diet changes can help drastically reduce the risk of chronic disease in middle age.

FINAL TIPS FOR A SUCCESSFUL FASTING MEAL PLAN

Great job! You're almost ready to begin your lifestyle change. Follow the steps given in this book carefully, and you'll soon feel full of energy, have better mental clarity, and you'll also lose weight without having to restrict calories severely or spend hours cooking and prepping food each day. As you have learned by now, some women succeed with fasting, and others give up. Indeed, keeping up with positive changes is difficult because you are doing something you're not used to. You're saying "no" to having a burger or a hotdog on the commute and instead deciding to invest more in healthy foods. However, this change also means that you won't be brushing your eating habits to the side, and you'll consciously invest time and effort into healthier eating.

For many women, regardless of their age, this seems like a futile investment. Why would you spend two hours shopping for healthy foods when you can use this time for anything else—work, learning, hobbies, or chores? If you think about it a bit more, a healthy diet is an investment. But the reason we start to feel like it's a waste of time and money is that we're failing to notice how much unhealthy eating costs in the long run. Think how much time you'll save when you become more energetic, and you're able to complete tasks more quickly. Think about the money you'll save on medications and treatments for preventable illnesses. Think about how your work and personal relationships improve once you're more vital, productive, and sharp-minded.

Finally, let go of the idea that investing time and effort in healthy eating is futile. You're securing yourself with decades of healthy, quality life, and you deserve to take better care of yourself. With that in mind, let's reflect on the importance of having a meal and everything a meal plan helps you with.

Clean Food Choices

The more you have to ask yourself, "What am I going to eat?" the greater the risk of settling for unhealthy food. A meal plan allows you to sit down and look at the exact foods that you wish to include in your diet. You can think about their macronutrient ratios and decide how to combine your foods so that you're within the scope of your balanced, low-carb, or keto reference. Without planning, your meals could easily have more carbs or fat than needed or healthy, which can potentially diminish the health effects and slow down fat burning.

Conscious Diet Decisions

You can adjust your intermittent fasting lifestyle for balanced, keto, and low carb eating. Here are the key differences in macronutrient ratios for these diets:

A balanced diet favors carbs (45-65%) but still allows plenty of protein (10-35%) and fat (20-35%) in your daily nutrition. For healthy weight maintenance, your net calories should equate to your daily calorie spending, which depends on your height, weight, and lifestyle. Even with intermittent fasting, weight loss should entail a slight calorie deficit. Almost all studies were done on the effects of the balanced diet signal success, given that meals are properly measured and that you eat 100-200 calories less than your average expenditure.

The keto diet, on the other hand, emphasizes fat (55-60%) over protein (30-35%), keeping the carbs at the very minimum (5-10%). Once you manage to get into ketosis, you'll start shedding weight like you wouldn't believe!

The low-carb diet lets you have fun with protein (40-50%) and fat (30-35%) while maintaining a low-carb intake (15-24%).

Organize Your Cooking and Grocery Shopping

Planning your meals also helps you decide how to cook and schedule, pre-making several meals at once. Pre-making meals helps prepare for busy days when you won't have the time to make your meals.

A plan sets you up for success because you know what foods you'll need for the week. This helps organize your shopping, and it makes it easier to abstain from eating during your fasting hours. Having enough healthy food at your disposal helps you get the nutrition that you need during your eating hours and reduces the chance of feeling an overly intense appetite while fasting.

Plan Meals You'll Love

A diet that works is one that allows you to eat the foods you like and in sufficient quantities so that you don't feel like you're starving. Now, think about your eating preference—do you wish for several smaller meals or fewer bigger meals? It's commonly recommended to have three main meals and two snacks if you prefer smaller meals scattered throughout the day. However, if you don't want to have five different meals, then your task is to distribute all of your recommended calories to three meals, without any snacking or treats before, afterward, and between. That's not easy, so think carefully about which eating schedule will work best for you.

Keep Your Diet Rich and Versatile

Make sure to have enough lean protein, as this will support your muscle tissue preservation. Planning helps get into the macronutrient distribution of the foods you like, which can make you realize that you can have far more than you initially thought without weight gain. However, your lean meat and healthy dairy should come without starchy side dishes and sauces.

Vegetables are low in net carbs, and they're packed with beneficial micronutrients that benefit your health and diet. However, the very mention of keto or low carb can make you feel like you're only allowed fat and meat. This isn't true. If you look at your daily calorie spending, you'll notice that you can have plenty of veggies and still stay within your selected carb limit.

If you wish to include carbs in your diet, go for whole vegetables instead of processed, sugary foods. You can enjoy sweet and regular potatoes, rice, carrots, cruciferous vegetables, and many more!

Healthy fats are important as well, and you have many options for healthy eating. You can enjoy olive oil, dairy, butter, cheeses, fatty fish, and other treats you like—as long as they're not processed. Stay away from toxic processed oils such as canola oil, palm oil, soybean oil, corn oil, etc.

CONCLUSION

Great work on learning the basics of intermittent fasting, and kudos for deciding to make a wholesome change in your life! If you still doubt your ability to follow through with a fasting lifestyle, relax. Your body is genetically wired to succeed in this process. All the weight loss and wellness tools are already in you, and that's the beauty of fasting. Fasting allows you to access your inner potential to harvest energy and nutrients from the gifts of nature that food is and then use those nutrients to replenish each tiny cell in your body. Isn't that amazing?

Whenever in doubt, simply recap what your eating and lifestyle habits looked like before and how different that is from what a human body is made of. Look back at women's lifestyles prior to the modern age, and you'll be fascinated by how strong and resilient they used to be. These women, who lived mainly from heavy labor and in much worse living conditions, enjoyed much more vitality and physical strength. Granted, the life spans weren't nearly as long as what we have today. But research that dove into the health of medieval women still confirmed that they had better physical and mental health than now. While technology, safety, and access to healthcare prolonged the lives of modern women, a lifestyle of stress and overindulgence in food that resulted had a devastating impact. Women globally struggle with obesity, cardiac issues, metabolic diseases, and diabetes more than ever. Even if we were to compare the numbers of malnourished with the obese, obesity would prevail.

The modern obesity epidemic can be attributed to one occurrence that's unique to modern history: constant insulin production in our bodies. Look back at the early 20th century, and you'll see that people's dietary and lifestyle habits were entirely different. Look even further into the past, and you'll realize that overconsumption of food is quite literally taking lives.

In this book, you learned that fasting is a simple yet effective tool to reverse the process of overproducing insulin and help your body get back into its natural balance. You learned that, in order to lose weight, you first need to address the problem of insulin resistance. Granted, medications help, and I am the first to tell you to go see a doctor and follow their instructions to the T. Yet not all medications in the world can help you if you don't make permanent lifestyle changes.

Intermittent fasting brings about the change you need. It teaches you to control your appetite and limit food intake to a select number of hours so that your body stops producing insulin and makes a metabolic shift to burning fatty supplies for energy. As you learned, this process can begin as early as three to four days into your lifestyle change.

As your body starts burning fat to fuel your body, you start losing weight steadily. Some women lose one to two pounds a month, and others drop even five to ten, depending on their physical activity and select diet regimen. As you learned in this book, you can reap many fasting benefits that boost the health of women in middle age.

The changes that happen in your body as a result of aging can, indeed, make it harder to slim down. Changes in hormonal balance also affect metabolism, and they can intervene with your sleep, which further affects weight loss. Moreover, your resting metabolism becomes slower, and you gradually lose muscle mass. Yet, not all is lost, and you still have plenty to look forward to when it comes to getting slim and fit. All the women you can learn about online are a living testament that female bodies can retain vitality and longevity regardless of age. But, you must work with the changes in your body and make your diet more nutrient-dense in order to burn fat and preserve muscle.

You also learned that there are many other benefits from fasting, all of them proven by research. You learned that fasting strengthens your immune system, cardiovascular health, cognitive sharpness, and mental resilience. It can help protect against life-threatening illnesses thanks to autophagy, a process in which your body metabolizes diseased cells to produce energy and then uses that energy to build vital cells. Isn't your body a miracle?

The first steps of successful fasting, as you learned, include thinking through your habits and lifestyle. You must commit to eating clean whole foods and give up sugary treats entirely. Then, you should look at how many calories you should be eating each day and select a diet regimen to follow. Your diet regimen may be Mediterranean, low carb, balanced, or keto. It doesn't matter as long as you make an educated decision that's based on the needs of your body.

Then, you can start fasting gradually. At first, you can practice 12-hour fasting and gradually reduce your eating times to six to eight hours. In this book, you also learned that there are more extreme methods of fasting that you can use weekly or monthly to give your metabolism an extra nudge and further strengthen and detoxify your body.

You also learned that having the right mindset for fasting is crucial for success. You can expect sugar cravings, mood changes, and different challenges with your body's detoxing process. At first, you might feel sluggish, irritable, and tired. Don't worry; all of this will pass if you persist in your efforts. Be sure to reflect on your habits of conditioned and habitual, even unconscious eating. Make sure that all of your decisions are based on your needs and not on circumstances and others' expectations. Don't be afraid to stand out, because the results will be more than worth the hassle! Within months, you'll feel like a whole new person.

Are you ready to start fasting? Take a few days to think about the best fasting method and start making your own weekly diet plans. Have you enjoyed your intermittent fasting guide? Don't forget to share your honest feedback on Amazon!

REFERENCES

Babio, N., Bulló, M., & Salas-Salvadó, J. (2009). Mediterranean diet and metabolic syndrome: the evidence. *Public Health Nutrition*, 12(9A), 1607–1617. https://doi.org/10.1017/S1368980009990449

Batitucci, G., Faria Junior, E. V., Nogueira, J. E., Brandão, C. F. C., Abud, G. F., Ortiz, G. U., Marchini, J. S., & Freitas, E. C. (2022). Impact of intermittent fasting combined with high-intensity interval training on body composition, metabolic biomarkers, and physical fitness in women with obesity. *Frontiers in Nutrition*, 9. https://doi.org/10.3389/fnut.2022.884305

Carb Manager (2022, February). *Intermittent fasting for women over 50: 7 tips for success*. Carb Manager. https://www.carbmanager.com/article/ygj3xheaaawus2xa/intermittent-fasting-for-women-over-50-7-tips-for/

Fung, J. (2019, April 25). *Your complete guide to intermittent fasting*. Diet Doctor. https://www.dietdoctor.com/intermittent-fasting

Galang, M. (2022, May 19). *What women over 50 should know about intermittent fasting*. Nutritious Life. https://nutritiouslife.com/eat-empowered/intermittent-fasting-wome

Ganesan, K., Habboush, Y., & Sultan, S. (2018). *Intermittent fasting: the choice for a healthier lifestyle*. Cureus, 10(7). https://doi.org/10.7759/cureus.2947

Harvard T.H. Chan. (2018, January 16). *Diet review: Mediterranean diet*. The Nutrition Source. https://www.hsph.harvard.edu/nutritionsource/healthy-weight/diet-reviews/mediterranean-diet/

Liu, H., Javaheri, A., Godar, R. J., Murphy, J., Ma, X., Rohatgi, N., ... & Diwan, A. (2017). Intermittent fasting preserves beta-cell mass in obesity-induced diabetes via the autophagy-lysosome pathway. *Autophagy*, 13(11), 1952-1968.

Mackenthun, A. (2021). The effects of intermittent fasting on type 2 diabetes. *Journal of Advanced Writing*, 2.

Mattson, M. P., et al. (2017). *Impact of intermittent fasting on health and disease processes.* Ageing Research Reviews, vol. 39, Oct. 2017, pp. 46–58, www.sciencedirect.com/science/article/pii/S1568163716302513, 10.1016/j.arr.2016.10.005.

Savanelli, M. C., Barrea, L., Macchia, P. E., Savastano, S., Falco, A., Renzullo, A., Scarano, E., Nettore, I. C., Colao, A., & Di Somma, C. (2017). Preliminary results demonstrating the impact of Mediterranean diet on bone health. *Journal of Translational Medicine,* 15(1). https://doi.org/10.1186/s12967-017-1184-x

Stanton, B. (2021). How does keto affect cholesterol? Carb Manager. https://www.carbmanager.com/article/yvwt8raaamyw6mtt/how-does-keto-affect-cholesterol/

Tamber, M. (2022, June 17). *Does intermittent fasting cause muscle loss?* Diet Doctor. https://www.dietdoctor.com/intermittent-fasting/muscle-loss

Walters, M. (2021, February 4). *Intermittent fasting for real people: Practical tips to eat on schedule.* Healthline. https://www.healthline.com/health/food-nutrition/intermittent-fasting-for-real-people-practical-tips-to-eat-on-schedule#tips

Well Org Team. (2019, July 2). 7 intermittent fasting tips and tricks for better results. Well.org. https://well.org/healthy-body/intermittent-fasting-results-tips/

Yin, W., Löf, M., Chen, R., Hultman, C. M., Fang, F., & Sandin, S. (2021). Mediterranean diet and depression: a population-based cohort study. *International Journal of Behavioral Nutrition and Physical Activity,* 18(1). https://doi.org/10.1186/s12966-021-01227-3